Demotic

VOLUME X

BY: TODD ANDREW ROHRER

iUniverse, Inc.
New York   Bloomington

Demotic

iUniverse books may be ordered through booksellers or by contacting:

iUniverse
1663 Liberty Drive
Bloomington, IN 47403
www.iuniverse.com
1-800-Authors (1-800-288-4677)

ISBN: 978-1-4401-8580-9 (pbk)
ISBN: 978-1-4401-8581-6 (ebook)

Printed in the United States of America

iUniverse rev. date:10/23/09

Demotic: noun: demotic script; planned written language.

The only doubt I have is whether I sit or stand on the fence.

8/30/2009 11:21:44 PM
[Genesis 11:1 And the whole earth was of one language, and of one speech.]

    This denotes before written language there was only one tongue and that was verbal language and it was an evolving language. Planned language denotes many rules and also sequence in order to use the written forms of this planned language. Evolving language denotes there was no right or wrong thing to say. This evolving language was simply verbal not written. So this comment is simply saying at one time there was only verbal communication and no written communication. One way to look at this is when a person meets someone who speaks a different language they are still able to communicate to a degree. So for example there is a person who speaks Spanish and a person who speaks English. If they were both trapped on an island they would figure out a way to communicate and once they did it would be a new kind of language or an evolving language. So the person who spoke English would use many English words thrown in with a few Spanish words they slowly started to learn so this is what "one speech" denotes. Where there is a will to communicate it will happen, so to speak. So in this regard planned written language has isolated people. Do you speak English? So a person who does not speak English will feel left out, so to speak. This encourages this left brain, seeing things in parts. The deeper meaning is the more planned languages one learns the more rules and sequencing one undertakes mentally and thus the more left brain dominate you become.

Left Brain = Sequential
Right Brain = Random Access

1

9/1/2009 10:30:59 PM

[Genesis 11:4 And they said, Go to, let us build us a city and a tower, whose top may reach unto heaven; and let us make us a name, lest we be scattered abroad upon the face of the whole earth.]

This is in relation to after man has gotten written language education or has eaten off the tree of knowledge. So the first comment suggests at one time there was only verbal language. This comment suggests after man invented written language they started to exhibit some different characteristics. Man became left brained and started seeing things in a physical perspective and thus their cerebral abilities started to dwindle. This tower denotes mankind started looking at physical ways to achieve satisfaction. They wanted to build a physical tower to reach heaven. This is because man went extreme left brain from learning written script language and they started to look at physical aspects more than cerebral aspects. So this comment is simply explaining the mental side effects written language started causing. Man forgot heaven is in the mind or is cerebral and started looking for heaven as a physical place instead of a state of mind. "And let us make us a name" denotes parts. Man started to label things and that is left brain. Man stopped seeing things as a whole so their right brain was veiled and their left brain in turn became dominate. "Lest we be scattered" denotes at one time man was scattered. Scattered denotes free or wandering as in hunters and gatherers. So this is simply showing how mankind mentally started changing after they started using written language, man started flocking together in separate groups known as cities. They started seeing parts and using labels and started becoming very physical based in their thoughts as opposed to seeing everything as a whole and being cerebral based in their thoughts. So there are some psychological contrast aspects as a result of learning sequential based written language.

The deeper meaning of a person trying to build a physical tower to reach heaven when heaven is right brain, which has been veiled because one has learned written language, is called vanity. So it is very vain to try to build a physical tower to reach heaven when in reality one has to do some mental fear conditioning to reach heaven,

2

unveil right brain after its been veiled inadvertently from learning written language. It is vanity to try to reach satisfaction in the physical world when satisfaction is between the ears it simply has to be unveiled after ones gets the "education."

[Genesis 15:1 After these things the word of the LORD came unto Abram in a vision, saying, Fear not, Abram: I am thy shield, and thy exceeding great reward.]

One has to do some serious mental fear not conditioning to reach "heaven". Physical things are not going to help one unveil right brain because it requires mental conditioning. Simply put it is all on the shoulders of each person who got this education to get their self out of that left brain dominate hell they are in. That's what the stone around the neck is or the yoke around the neck relates to.

[Genesis 11:5 And the LORD came down to see the city and the tower, which the children of men builded.]

So the Lords or the ones who negated or did not get the written language and thus were of sound mind came and saw this city and tower which denotes civilization, which the children of men built. So "men" in this comment is an insult. It is like saying the serpent. The children of the serpent built this city and tower which shows they got the written language education and started to show some mental changes and one of these changes was they started to settle. They stopped wandering or living in the wilderness.

So this is a separation of normal human beings who did not get the education or negated the effects of the left brain conditioning education and were called Lords as in Lords of the mind or of sound mind, and men which were ones who got the education and thus were of the serpent in relation to mental characteristics. What I see is human beings, Lords, who were not extreme left brained and were of sound mind were making observations of these strange acting human beings who did get the "education" and the Lords named them men.

3

So the Lords are saying "Look what the men are making their children do." This is very complex because the whole reason these "men" needed to start building houses and shelters is because in extreme left brain one is very susceptible to being irritated easily. One in extreme left brain gets cold very easily, gets hot very easily and these things bother them very much. The Lords are asking, "Why aren't these men sleeping out under the stars like we have been for thousands of years?". "Why do they need to build all these shelters called cities?" "What is wrong with living in the wilderness, we have done it for thousands of years and as long as we can remember?" So the point is, this written education made "men" so left brained they had to start doing things to compensate for this unsound mental state learning written language put them in.

So "men" learned written language and then all of these problems started popping up. So then the "men" had to start trying to fix all these perceived problems but in reality these problems were a symptom they had learned written language and it made them very left brained and thus of unsound mind, so they were not real problems in an absolute form, they were only perceived to be problems by the "men" with unsound minds. The deepest meaning of this is the "men" took a perfectly good mind of a child and determine they had to "fix it" by teaching that child written language, they could not leave well enough alone. That's the whole problem, they determined this written language would fix a child that is already perfectly mentally balanced and in turn they sent that child into extreme left brain and in fact mentally ruined that child. This is why education is based on a lie.

Education determines children are not mentally balanced unless they get written education and that is a lie because in fact written education makes a child mentally unbalanced or extreme left brain and thus veils the complex right brain if not applied properly. Simply put the remedy "fear not" to counter act the written language education is so harsh, a person is better off not getting written language education because once they do they simply may never be able to get back to sound mind because the fear not remedy taken to the full measure is in fact mental suicide. Go ask a psychologist if mental suicide or fear not is safe then you will understand you may be doomed mentally to where you are at. One has the literally die mentally and what makes it even harder is one cannot resist or fight back or "try to save their self".

[Luke 17:33 ... and whosoever shall lose his life shall preserve it.]

This is why if one got the education they are in a serious pickle. There is no human being on the left that is going to say "Yes it is mentally wise to put yourself in a situation where you think you are going to die and then allow it." That's mental suicide. To ones on the left that is crazy talk. To ones of sound mind that is truth. So one is in a situation they are going to have to think for their self and ignore what the "experts" who are in extreme left brain suggest. Simply put the ones on the left are of unsound mind so their advice is unsound. Do you trust what a "lord" says is right or what a man says is right because they are going to be opposite suggestions or contrary suggestions. Ones on the left will say:

[Luke 17:33 ... seek to save his life...;.]

The ones on the left will say "Seek to save your life, Do not go to a cemetery alone to fight your fears away." You do not have to ask the ones on the left what they will say because that is what they will say. You are going to have to think for yourself.

That's the price one has to pay because when one was still mentally developing an adult forced them to get hardcore sequential education and thus made their mind extreme left brained. I always had the impression the adults were suppose to protect the children but now I understand that is the biggest lie in the universe.

Suffer the children is the only truth I understand. There are only two teams in all reality. The team who mentally rapes children and the team who tries to assist the children back to sound mind after the initial team mentally rapes them. There are no other teams, into infinity. The team that mentally rapes never loses because they have all the weapons and all the laws on their side that allows them to mentally rape children. They never ever lose. The other team always loses. They can never counter act how many children the initial team mentally rapes ever. So you have two choices, you can stay on the team that never loses or join the team that never wins and in order to join the team that never wins you have to have no ego or emotional capacity because they are never going to win. In order to join the team that never wins you have to commit mental suicide to break out of the extreme left brain state you were educated into as a child. This is the only choice there is to make in life. All other choices are simply foolish details. One team has all the luxuries and one team gets annihilated game after game. It seems pretty reasonable and smart to join the luxurious teams doesn't it? One might suggest that luxurious team is irresistible.

[Genesis 11:6 And the LORD said, Behold, the people is one, and they have all one language; and this they begin to do: and now nothing will be restrained from them, which they have imagined to do.]
    "The people is one" denotes the people did see everything as one thing and that is a right brain characteristic, seeing everything as a whole. When a person is of sound mind they have left and right hemisphere equal in power so one sees things as a whole because right brain is dominate over left brain. This is complex but when the mind is 50/50 left and right, right brain is the more complex and the most powerful of the two hemispheres so ones tends to show many symptoms of right brain like seeing things as a whole, complexity in thoughts, paradox, and creativity and of course ambiguity or doubt but one is still able to use sequence but not see things are parts very well, like using a comma is a judgment and it's also a symptom of seeing parts of a sentence. So one will not be very good at written language anymore, it will take effort because the mind will not be able to stay on topic very well, one will say things that appear odd to the ones on the left because they speak in random access thoughts as much as speak in sequential thoughts.
    "They all have one language" denotes verbal communication. "and this they begin to do" means and now things have changed because of this written language, the tree of knowledge. "Now nothing will be restrained from them", this is complex. When mind is sound one is mentally neutral or one is not a very good judge because one has right brain unveiled so they do not see parts but

the whole. So they are mentally in nothingness. "Nothing will be restrained from them" means they will lose this neutral state of mind. So this is explaining the mental change and psychology of people after they started learning this written language and going left brained to unsound state of mind, they started to be judges. One example is, when a teacher gives a student an F for misspelling words on a spelling test, that teacher is judging that student and forcing that student to learn to sequence letters properly to spell words "properly" so they are punishing that child with an F, and that child is forced to become left brained which is sequential based thoughts, or they understand they will be punished by their parents for failing that class.

It's essentially carrot and stick mental brainwashing. A child knows if they do not perform in the education, which is sequencing and thus turning their mind to extreme left brain, they will be punished harshly by their parents. One might suggest they are all in one killing the minds of the children because they no longer have the mental ability to understand what they do, so they know not what they do.

[Genesis 11:7 Go to, let us go down, and there confound their language, that they may not understand one another's speech.]

So people started inventing many different written languages and they became separated by that written language. This is an indication of left brain seeing things as parts. This is the start of separation of mankind itself. One group says "We use this written language and you do not so we are different or better than you." So then mankind had a reason to create nations. The nations are simply people who speak the same written language. "That they may not understand one another's speech." is saying this is where separations from seeing people as a whole which is right brain or one of sound mind as in 50/50 left and right brain, to people seeing parts which is a left brain extreme trait. So essentially this chapter is explaining how the learning of written language altered the people minds, made them left brain dominate and in turn changed how they acted on all levels.

9/1/2009 5:24:26 PM- Not that I ever get off topic but, Socrates is a very interesting contrast to this religious take so to speak. I think Socrates tried to keep it real as he tried to avoid the supernatural suggestions, of course he still got slaughtered by the sane but it was an example of ones who wake up try many strategies to reach the sane. A philosopher is simply a thinker and thinker denotes one who is very cerebral based. So a "true philosopher" as Socrates suggested does not fear death. That is exactly what is said about Jesus, "He defeated death.", as in his fear of death. They were both telling the truth. Ones on the left see many parts so they perhaps would never make that connection because one in extreme left brain is not very good at detecting patterns, that is a right brain characteristic. Right brain is not concerned with rules in these pattern detections. What that means is one in left brain would "defeat" their self in trying to make connection between Socrates, Moses, Buddha, Jesus, Mohammed because this would break all their preconceived rules of what they assume.

Right brain detects patterns and is not assuming there are rules. Right brain it is only concerned with patterns. So one on the left would say Socrates was in no way like Jesus, Moses, Buddha or Mohammed but in fact he was saying the exact same thing they were. So when right brain is unveiled after the "curse" is broken one becomes very open minded but that is because right brain is very good at detecting patterns and not so worried about rules in detection of the patterns.

[Proverbs 4:6 Forsake her not, and she shall preserve thee: love her, and she shall keep thee.] [Luke 17:33 … and whosoever shall lose his life shall preserve it.]

Preserve. This is saying the same thing in both of these comments but the sane may not detect the pattern. The fountain of youth is simply suggesting preserve.

[Genesis 19:26 But his wife looked back from behind him, and she became a pillar of salt.]

Salt is a preservative. The reality of these ancient texts and many of these ancient parables is they are all saying the same thing over and over in attempting to try to make a convincing argument to the sane but the catch is, the ones one the left have right brain veiled so they hear but do not understand. This is what all the ancient texts are saying through and through.

Written language did some things to your mind and made it unsound and made you have much fear as a side effect. One has to do some serious hardcore fear conditioning and silence that fear to a major degree to go back to sound mind. If one does not do that they will be unsound in mind and one will act strange and not have full mental capacity.

So Proverbs is saying do not forsake right brain and apply fear not and she will preserve thee. That means one will not have all of these unhealthy mental and physical aspects. Over eating, stress, confusion, depression, fear, nervous so they will be more healthy and thus preserved and it's much more complex than that but that's a shallow explanation. Then the next one is saying the same thing with the remedy attached, so it is an adaptation to the proverbs comment. It is saying do not try to run for help and save yourself when you are in a situation of perceived death and you will unveil right brain and break the curse of written language, left brain to an extreme, and that will give you these preservation aspects back.

So the comment just before the woman turned to salt is important to understand. Why did she turn to salt? Here is why.

[Gen 19:24 Then the LORD rained upon Sodom and upon Gomorrah brimstone and fire from the LORD out of heaven;

Gen 19:25 And he overthrew those cities, and all the plain, and all the inhabitants of the cities, and that which grew upon the ground.

Gen 19:26 But his wife looked back from behind him, and she became a pillar of salt.

Gen 19:27 And Abraham gat up early in the morning to the place where he stood before the LORD:

28 And he looked toward Sodom and Gomorrah, and toward all the land of the plain, and beheld, and, lo, the smoke of the country went up as the smoke of a furnace.]

The Lords or tribes were burning these new cities created by the ones who got the written language education. Abraham was burning them to the ground. They were abnormal these cities. Abraham was trying to stop the spread of this curse. Moses got his Exodus attack strategy from Abraham. The cities were not normal they were abnormal. Human beings didn't live in these things called cities and everyone in these cities were mentally unsound and acting very strange in contrast to the Lords or the ones who either broke the "curse" which is extreme left brain dominate from learning the written language, or the ones who never got the curse, education.

[Genesis 11:5 And the LORD came down to see the city and the tower, which the children of men builded.]

So in Chapter 11 the Lords saw these cities and in Chapter 19 they started burning them to the ground. Everyone in them was mentally cursed because they got the written language. Abraham and all the others were trying to stop this cursed "man" that started doing weird things after they got the education.

The American Indians tried to do the exact same thing. They tried to stop these "cursed" things from destroying everything in their path. So the ones on the left were curses and destroying everything in their path and the Lords were trying to stop them. Granted they failed but none the less they did try. They tried and failed to stop the curse and they called that curse "man". The curse is all relative to the unsound mind a person is in when they are educated with this written language called demotic. It is a subtle transition. It is nearly not noticeable when one is getting the education and this is because one gets rewards.

In a child's case their mind is not even fully developed when they start getting the education so a child is never even able to develop mentally before they are conditioned into this extreme left brain. So a child is punished for not getting the education or doing poor at the education by both the teacher and the parents and a child is rewarded for doing well at the education. So a child is rewarded for veiling their complex right brain by their parents, teacher, and also society.

It is perhaps too sinister for the sane to even grasp this because one who is mentally raped tends to sympathize with the one who raped them. One who gets this education has based their whole existence on the fact society would never do such a thing to them and when it is suggested that is in fact is exactly what has happened, they will deny that reality. The ones on the left have the powerhouse unnamable right brain veiled so they perhaps cannot do the proper mental processing to put all this together. One could easily suggest with this kind of sinister aspect that perhaps a supernatural aspect is involved but one could also make the case that this left brain conditioning is so subtle and appears like a wise decision so it simply goes undetected.

[Genesis 3:6 And when the woman saw that the tree was good for food, and that it was pleasant to the eyes, and a tree to be desired to make one wise, she took of the fruit thereof, and did eat, and gave also unto her husband with her; and he did eat.]

So written language looked like a good way to get educated. It looked very nice to the eyes, the letters are pretty and some written languages are very pretty to the eyes. It looked like a good way to keep records of events and then one could get wise from reading those records. It was a very convincing Trojan horse. Certainly nothing with all these great aspects could do anything bad to the mind. So then one may understand it was quite an irresistible fruit on that tree. All these details will never change one fact. One is going to have to go through the fire to break the mental curse. All of these words will not wake you up fully. This will wake you up fully.

[Luke 17:33 ... and whosoever shall lose his life shall preserve it.]

That comment is saying one has to commit mental suicide. One has to go sit in a situation they perceive they will die and then not try to save their self. I would suggest a very scary place. The Buddhists suggest meditate in a cemetery at night. One on the left is not going to be mediating they are going to be scared out of their mind and they will perhaps run like the wind. Here is what I did and you will

11

see it was an accident. I took a handful of pills to kill myself and when I was very sick I thought "I should call for help" then I thought "No I want to die" so I did not save myself and thus I preserved it, right brain and thus broke the curse, extreme left brain dominate state. The scary place technique is advisable.

We all got the education because it's a law we had to get the education so dwelling on that is meaningless. That aspect is not going to wake you up. One is simply going to have to scare their self to death and then not try to save their self. Perhaps the best way to go about it is to treat this event one has to go through as a suicide. One is going to go to a very scary place and they are going to die so they should make peace with their friends and get their things in order because they may not come out alive, that's the mindset. I know nothing about meditation. I did not wake up because I meditated. I woke up from earnestly trying to kill myself and when my mind said I was certainly going to die I did not try to save myself or call for help. That's all I know and that is also exactly what this means:

[Luke 17:33 … and whosoever shall lose his life shall preserve it.]

One is going to have to achieve this mental state called meek and humility and submission. One wants to wake up the full measure. There is no point in waking up halfway. One is going to be hot and not cold or lukewarm. There is nothing in all existence more important than this one act and if one does not understand that they clearly are not thinking clearly. There is no ghost that is going to kill you but you have to be in such an isolated place your mind tells you one certainly will or it won't work. Simply put, one has to look at Medusa's head and perhaps none of the ones on the left want to do that voluntarily. This all is relative to one thing. Powers that be, are you certain this written language you are pushing on everyone by law is worth it? Powers that be, you know not what you do. Powers that be, you put people mentally in a situation that is nearly impossible for them to get out of. Vox ut exsisto , vos precor ut vestri meretricis everto ut EGO operor non adepto tepidus sursum.

In case one is wondering what Sodom and Gomorrah is, it is every single city in the world because ever single city in the world teaches written language and they all exhibit the exact same symptom that Sodom and Gomorrah exhibited. Simply put.

[Genesis 18:26 And the LORD said, If I find in Sodom fifty righteous within the city, then I will spare all the place for their sakes.]

You are not going to find 50 people who have broken the curse to the full measure in any city in the world. There might only be one in the whole world. The complexity is, all of these wise beings in these ancient texts had to wake up which means they got the education. That is very complex because one who never gets the education has no contrast to how they were and how they are. Simply put they never were "mentally dead" so they don't know what it was like.

So the tribes needed Moses because Moses was in "civilization" and then he woke up and lead the tribes against civilization. Essentially he understood what this written language did to him. Jesus also woke up so he got the written language. Mohammed got the written language and he had to wake up. This contrast of being in the 'curse" and then waking up explains what "Vengeance is mine" means.

[Psalms 99:8 Thou answeredst them, O LORD our God: thou wast a God that forgavest them, though thou tookest vengeance of their inventions.]

Inventions like written language (Demotic) and Math. Both are very sequential based and have many rules and that is left brain.

[Exodus 32:19 And it came to pass, as soon as he came nigh unto the camp, that he saw the calf, and the dancing: and Moses' anger waxed hot, and he cast the tables out of his hands, and brake them beneath the mount.]

One might suggest when I hear the powers that be boasting about the children they are going to educate with their great invention my anger starts wax hot because the powers that be certainly are proud of their whore demotic. This is why the tablets or laws do not matter when the powers that be start everyone's life off by mentally raping them. Who cares about laws when you start getting mentally raped when you are about seven. Tribuo sanus operor ignoro quis brain

13

muneris est quoniam they sentio retardation est brain muneris , sic is est universa. I am blessed that no one can understand anything I say ever. - 7:15:30 PM

7:26:39 PM – So this comment:

[Genesis 19:26 But his wife looked back from behind him, and she became a pillar of salt.]

The above comment simply means the Lords burned down the cities and then this woman saw what they did and she became a "believer" and applied fear not and woke up and was preserved mentally thus turned to salt, preserved. I understand the sane have not understood one of these sentences in 2500 years, not even one sentence. Not even close, they are clueless.

9/2/2009 4:37:52 AM – Essentially the Abraham and Isaac method, fear not and [Luke 17:33 … and whosoever shall lose his life shall preserve it.] and "Meek shall inherit the earth" and submit to fear are all along the lines of mental suicide, except they are suggesting mental suicide and not literal suicide but it is a very fine line.

[Luke 17:33 … and whosoever shall lose his life shall preserve it.]
    That looks very much like suicide to me but it is really mental suicide. The sane are afraid of a bad hair cut so no wonder they slaughtered all these wise beings. The ones on the left push or teach this written language which veils a person's complex right brain then when the wise ones try to suggest a remedy so one can regain a sound mind they get slaughtered by the sane because what they suggest as a remedy sounds very "unsafe". That certainly sounds like the actions of a demon, good thing I don't detect supernatural. Haud admiratio EGO have haud mores quod haud ordo , EGO sum trying ut defero per mental abominations. I am not a fish that is concerned about their attempts at sequential elementary logic. Simply put, my ways are not their ways, my days are not their days.- 4:45:14 AM

6:54:22 AM – [Genesis 18:20 And the LORD said, Because the cry of Sodom and Gomorrah is great, and because their sin is very grievous;]
    The seven deadly sins are simply mental characteristics of ones who got the education and did not apply fear not. Very grievous denotes their mental state is able to achieve these "sins" for a very long time because the powerhouse right brain is veiled so they tend to be slothful in their thoughts. They can hold a grudge for a lifetime in contrast to one with right brain unveiled who can ponder through that grudge swiftly which denotes to one who has an overall neutral state of mind. Grievous also denotes they force the education on the minds of children and so they mentally ruin a child and veil the unnamable power of right brain so they sin against the unnamable, and that is an unforgivable sin because once a child's mind is

15

ruined when this education is not applied properly, the right brain powerhouse is veiled, the fruits of that child are ruined and so anyone who encourages this can never be forgiven, ever, into infinity.

Mental suicide is the domain of the wise and beyond the limits of the fearful.

[Mark 3:29 - But he that shall blaspheme against the Holy Ghost hath never forgiveness, but is in danger of eternal damnation:]

Once the right brain, unnamable power, is veiled, one is doomed because they are left with the sequential stupid left brain to try and live and that's not going to happen because one needs both hemispheres active to have a chance at life so they are dammed and if one encourages that on others, they are dammed.

What are you? - http://www.youtube.com/watch?v=YNaTQzLb4NI

Music creation is simply patterns or pattern creation. This pattern creation is relative to right brain so many musical artists tend to use drugs to unveil right brain and thus the pattern aspect of the mind is unleashed and then music creation becomes very easy or effortless. Birds for example make many different "songs" and this is because their right brain is unveiled so they can make very complicated sounding "songs" but from their perspective it is simply patterns. So music itself is not really music it is simply patterns. Spoken language itself is essentially verbal patterns. Very good orators are adept at making words fall into patterns and these patterns are what are pleasing to a crowd. Anyone can arrange words but a poet can rearrange them. It is not what one says it is how one says it and that is the pattern. The pattern of what one says is what makes what one says effective or not and patterns are relative to right brain. Creativity is relative to right brain. Both pattern detection ability and creativity are the bottom line to everything. With enough creativity and pattern detecting ability one can perhaps solve any problem. The pattern is detected and the creativity is used to adjust patterns or come up with solutions so when the right brain is veiled problems become very hard to solve.

When right brain is veiled living one's life becomes very difficult. When right brain is veiled easy problems become difficult problems. Difficulty creates frustration and this frustration creates a mental sense of "life is too hard". So the veiling of the right brain which is what written language education does, simply turns an easy life into a huge problem that seems to be very difficult to solve.- 9:43:51 AM

9/3/2009 7:08:20 AM – I will give my take on the story of the good Samaritan just off the top of my head and I will cover it in detail in a later volume perhaps. The one who is lying in the road represents the ones who got the education and no one wants to get near that person, because they have to go up against the powers that be first, which are the ones who push the education and do not suggest the remedy thus leaving people mentally unbalanced. So the Samaritan is the one who decides to go up against the powers that be, that puts the people mentally in the road dying. Many pass up that test because they want to save their self. Simply put they are afraid of the taskmaster. Anyone who tries to help that person in the road is going to be slaughtered by the taskmaster because the taskmaster is all about keeping the people dumb, fearful and mentally unbalanced so the taskmaster can easily control his slaves with fear tactics.

There is no way anyone is going to convince the taskmaster to apply the fear conditioning remedy after they force the left brain education on the people because the people would be far to sound minded and then the taskmaster would lose all of his powers or control and thus power over his slaves. So the good Samaritan story is all relative to the comment.

[John 15:13 - Greater love hath no man than this, that a man lay down his life for his friends.]

So in perspective, the wise ones tried to assist their friends and let them know what the mental side effects of the education is and tried to suggest a remedy so one is not robbed of their complex right brain and thus their naturally given heightened awareness and the taskmaster slaughtered them all. So you make sure you think very carefully before you apply the fear not remedy because once you do you join the team that never wins and that denotes you join the lambs to slaughter team.

The wise beings were fully aware of their fate long before they were slaughtered. This appears to be some supernatural aspect but I understand that is just a symptom of one who has right brain unveiled. One is able to think in random access thoughts so they can reach the eventuality or end conclusion swiftly. One example of

18

this is when Jesus was in the wilderness praying and trying to see if he could avoid his fate. This is what heightened awareness is all about. One is aware of the future or the end result not because they are supernatural perhaps but because they can think many moves ahead which is contrary to one who is extreme left brained who can only think in sequential thought, left brain is sequential based like language is and so one is mentally slothful in contrast.

Left brain thinking is sequential so one can only think one move ahead. When right brain is unveiled one can think all the moves ahead that are required, and do that at lightning speed. The sane perhaps cannot grasp that but the ones who are awake understand that naturally or without anyone having to tell them that. The complexity is one is aware of what the end conclusion is, but they have no fear, so they are not able to really be scared away, they just take it like troopers.

They simply become this:
[John 15:13 - Greater love hath no man than this, that a man lay down his life for his friends.]

There is a deep complexity to this situation. The ones on the left hear but do not understand the complexity because right brain is complexity and theirs is veiled, so complexity is beyond their mental ability, until the apply the fear not conditioning. The ones on the left read these ancient texts and everything is over their head. Here is a good example of this.

Moses battled the ones on the left and freed the people and he took them to the wilderness or away from the cities. So Moses tried to make everything as it was or show people we are supposed to live in the "wild" so to speak. So Moses tried to deny the city life all together and tried to just restore living in the wilderness. Jesus did not get far enough to attempt to free the people because he was deemed a threat by the taskmaster and taken care of swiftly. Jesus was deemed a terrorist and a threat to the taskmaster so he never got very far in his Exodus plans. Mohammed adjusted his strategy and this is relative to the fact he came a thousand years after Moses. Mohammed did not try to free people and bring them back to the wilderness because he was aware it was far too late for that so

Mohammed tried to take the cities and adapt to the city life and still educate people but also apply the fear not remedy or submit to fear.

So the ones on the left assume Mohammed tried to take everyone "backwards" in progression so to speak but in reality Moses tried to negate or deny the city invention and Abraham simply burned the cities to the ground. Mohammed adapted to the cities it and Abraham simply burned the cities to the ground completely.

So Moses freed the people and tried to bring them back to the wilderness and Mohammed looked at the cities as acceptable and just tried to use that invention and tried to suggest submit to fear needs to be applied and the cities cannot be taken away and they are not the problem.

It is the mental state written language education leaves one in, that is the problem. This is a good example of how the ones on the left have everything backwards. Simply put, their minds are unsound because of twelve years of left brain indoctrination and then they are not told to apply the remedy to revert back to sound mind, which is fear not or fear conditioning. Everything in the ancient texts is over their head because their mind has the complex hemisphere veiled, everything. The ones on the left cannot even grasp Moses, Jesus and Mohammed were all on the same exact page. They perhaps can never grasp that into infinity. The ones who are awake understand the common thread of those three wise beings of the west without effort.

So one thousand years or more years before Mohammed this is what was done to this new invention cities.

[Gen 19:24 Then the LORD rained upon Sodom and upon Gomorrah brimstone and fire from the LORD out of heaven;]

The cities were burned to the ground by the "lords" and then Mohammed simply adapted to the reality the cities were acceptable or he adapted to the city reality. This is complex because perhaps the "lords" assumed the cities were the problem and if they burned them the problem would go away. This is indicated by this comment.

[Genesis 18:26 And the LORD said, If I find in Sodom fifty righteous within the city, then I will spare all the place for their sakes.]

The reality is, the cities were a symptom that the written education had made people very left brained. The cities were not what were making people left brained. This of course may make it seem like the wise ones in the Torah did not understand the problem but they did understand the problem. The wise ones were trying strategies to stop the spread of the curse because the ones who had the curse did not have the mental ability to grasp they were in fact mentally cursed after they learned the written language and did not apply the remedy, fear not.

Simply put it is impossible to convince the sane not to use written language and math so the next best thing was to just burn down their cities and wipe them out.

[Genesis 19:25 And he overthrew those cities, and all the plain, and all the inhabitants of the cities, and that which grew upon the ground.]

All the inhabitants means they wiped then all out and their cities in an attempt to make the problem go away but in reality written language had already spread all over the world, everyone was doing it so there was no way to stop it, so they understood total extermination of anyone who gets the education was a valid strategy. Even today, if there is say an apartment complex where for example a rare very contagious fatal form of a disease breaks out, like some rare form of rabies, they quarantine the entire building and no one comes out alive. So these wise being tries to stop the spread of this disease called left brain extreme caused by learning demotic and they failed, look at the world, but they gave it one hell of a shot. They tried the best they could but they were just human beings and once one get the neurosis caused by learning this sequential based invention they are pretty much done for anyway, mentally speaking.

[Genesis 3:14 And the LORD God said unto the serpent, Because thou hast done this, thou art cursed above all cattle, and above every beast of the field; upon thy belly shalt thou go, and dust shalt thou eat all the days of thy life:]

So the ones on the left could not grasp they were inadvertently mentally cursed above all cattle because they got the education and did not apply fear not as the remedy and what is even a deeper

21

reality is they still do not get it even today. They perhaps never will understand that into infinity because they are cursed mentally. "Shall eat all the days of their life" denotes they are perhaps cursed forever and ever. The complexity is once they get the education they go extreme left brained and then they have this anomaly called fear in their mind and the remedy is condition away from fear but they will not do that because they think fear is a valuable asset on one level and then on another level they listen to the fearful left brain intuition as if it is a true intuition when in reality is the deceiver or deceptive intuition. That is why when it comes right down the full measure, fear conditioning is essentially mental suicide:

[Luke 17:33 … and whosoever shall lose his life shall preserve it.]

The sane perhaps cannot do it because it appears unsafe. It appears like they may lose their life so they never preserve it, which mean unveiling right brain. So the curse is they have the fear from the education and to break the curse they have to face their greatest fear and they will never do that because their deceptive left brain intuition will not allow them to. I am blessed no one can understand anything I say ever.

[John 15:13 Greater love hath no man than this, that a man lay down his life for his friends.

John 15:14 Ye are my friends, if ye do whatsoever I command you.]

This is a deep comment because it is suggesting this "us against them" aspect. First this is Jesus sayings do what I suggest and then you will be my friend so it is also saying if you do not do what I suggest you are my adversary. So it is important to understand what Jesus was commanding. Jesus was commanding the covenant which is the only way to break the curse which is fear not or fear conditioning, as suggested by Abram at least five hundred years earlier.

[Genesis 15:1 After these things the word of the LORD came unto Abram in a vision, saying, Fear not, Abram: I am thy shield, and thy exceeding great reward.]

It is important to look at this fear not conditioning on a larger scale than just the western world. In Buddhism there is a practice where one goes to a cemetery and mediates at night alone. That is fear not or fear conditioning. The deeper meaning of what Abraham suggests is, he would not know the remedy unless he got the education first and then broke the curse accidentally so to speak. One who does not get the education has no need to apply fear not because they are of sound mind. One who does get the education cannot tell they are of unsound mind. The only way to discover one was "cursed" is to apply fear not.

Only in that situation can one have the contrast of how they were and how they are now and then figure out what happened. So the comment by Abraham is simply saying he had the accident and in time figured out he applied fear not conditioning the full measure. One cannot figure out the remedy unless they first get the education. The accident is so rare that there is this huge gap between these wise beings.

Buddha did not eat for 39 or 43 days and then had his accident and went out of his way to suggest, do not try to conditioning away fear by starving because you probably will starve to death, just go to a cemetery and mediate to lose fear of death. It is much safer that way and it perhaps just as effective. This is all relative to the reality this is not about physical things it is about psychology or a mental conditioning. That of course makes everything more complex. One has to mentally perceive they will die and then not fight it which is exactly what this means:

[Luke 17:33 … and whosoever shall lose his life shall preserve it.]

So this is another aspect of the curse that is perhaps the reason this curse has plagued mankind for so long. The education is easy to go into. It pleasing to look at and it appears it makes one wise.

[Genesis 3:6 And when the woman saw that the tree was good for food, and that it was pleasant to the eyes, and a tree to be desired to make one wise,....]

And then it goes even deeper because it has this string of wealth or money attached to it. So a person is in a position this education looks like a beautiful Trojan horse. The education can never have any bad mental side effects ever. That's also part of the curse. The education is too good to be true so everyone takes a big bite off that apple. That's is understood but the reality is once one takes a bite off that apple they have to pay the ferryman to get back to sound mind, and the ferryman's price is a price few can afford, a person has to not fear even though they have tons of fear. One has to commit mental suicide and that means they have to deny what that fear based left brain it is telling them is real, to run from a perceived life threatening situation. One is in a position they have to apply this fear not remedy their self but they will perhaps not want to do that because their left brain is telling them it would be life threatening to sit that cemetery all night alone in the dark with no chance to get help. But there are some who will mentally look at it like this:

[Mark 1:18 And straightway they forsook their nets, and followed him.]

They will look at it like there is nothing more important in the universe than to go for the gold so to speak. These are called seekers. They will rush to the most scary cemetery instantly and they will get [Genesis 15:1 ... exceeding great reward.], which is simply they will unveil the complex right brain and find mental life after their trial by fire, so to speak.

Some who are awake suggest perhaps it is best if one is a certain age they should just not worry about waking up. I beg to differ. Even if one is old, once they achieve consciousness time will be so silenced one day will seem like a very long time so even recovering at a very old age can make the life they have left last for a very long time. One might suggest one day is like a thousand years, so I will suggest it is never too late to wake up. One has nothing to lose and everything to gain.

The reality about the fear conditioning is it only takes one second. To clarify. One is mentally in a position they perceive their death is imminent and then they mentally accept that and let go, and that takes one second. It is simply a thought. Getting to that point is the part that needs to be thought out but it is perhaps rather easy to do since most on the left are afraid of their own shadow, so to speak.

I have spoken to ones on the left who suggest they would not go a cemetery at night because it does not scare them and so they would just be bored. I can only humbly suggest they are perhaps not using creativity. They are perhaps thinking about a city cemetery with lots of light and lots of cars driving by. I am suggesting the very old cemeteries out in the middle of nowhere and without a light to be seen. I am suggesting they have a friend drop them off over night. I am suggesting they bring no possible way to get help or get away if something happens as in ghosts. They will quickly respond with "That might be dangerous and perhaps deadly." And I humbly respond, "That's the whole point. You have to defeat death."

And they respond with "That is crazy." And I respond with "Perhaps." - 9:44:14 AM

9/4/2009 7:21:08 AM – I certainly get mocked a lot when I suggest this fear not concept and ironically I get mocked the most in religious chat rooms. Everything comes down to a few simple realities. I had an accident and lost my fear. That altered my mind. That denotes my mind was not in a natural state for a reason. So I accidentally lost my fear and it opened up my mind and now I am capable of extreme concentration and I can understand many things I could not understand for forty years. If you doubt that I am telling the truth then you need to experiment and prove me wrong.

If you mock what I say and do not even experiment with what I suggest then you are perhaps beyond help. If you experiment with what I suggest and it alters your mind then you are going to understand that this entire society mentally rapes children with their written language and math education because this entire society of earth perhaps does not have the brain function to understand what those two sequential based inventions do to the mind.

This is why it is important the sane never speak of morals because they are complicit in the mental raping of children and ruining their minds and I was one of them. I do not really care about what you say about what I say, because the last I checked you got mentally raped also and that means you are not really capable of this aspect called thinking clearly until you work on that log of fear in your eye. EGO operor non have quisquam in meus pars quod ut est bonus quoniam EGO operor non postulo quisquam in meus pars ut tracto vos.- 7:32:57 AM

10:09:30 AM – I spoke to some people in a chat room and explained the tree of knowledge and the remedy and I understand they understood what I was saying but then they go back to their ways like this fear not remedy is just not important. They understand the principle of what I suggest but their minds are unable to apply it. They forget about it right after I suggest it. They perceive their mental state is normal. I tell them I am an accident and I lost my fear accidentally and now everything mentally is different and they cannot compute that. They say they understand but then they say that the fear conditioning aspect sounds scary and then they just forget about it. This whole education invention has ruined people minds to such an extreme they cannot even think. So the powers that be suggest I should follow their laws even after I understand they rape people mentally as children and I was one of them. They perceive I acknowledge the suggestions of a rapist. Le seul commentaire que j'ai pour l'oppresseur est tes jours sont comptés. - 10:19:04 AM

2:25:38 PM – Fear hinders concentration and makes one confused and thus fearful.

6:54:33 PM – The ancient texts, the Torah the New Testament and the Quran are a paradox.

All three texts contain methods to save civilization.
All three texts contain methods to defeat civilization.

These ancient texts on one hand contain the psychological methods for negating the written languages mental side effects: fear not; lose your life mentally to preserve it(the mind) and submit to fear.

On the other hand the texts also list methods for dealing with the sane. The Torah has many examples of ways to fight against the sane. Jesus said he agreed with Moses or the Torah so he was in sync with those methods which had a lot to do with why the sane killed him swiftly.

The ancient texts main goal perhaps is to explain how a person who gets the education and has a veiled right brain as a result, can get back to a sound state of mind as in 50/50 left and right brain.

The next goal is how to deal with the ones who get the education and do not apply the fear not remedy because if they are left unchecked they will destroy the entire planet and its ecosystem and thus doom everyone. So the sane keep publishing these ancient texts that are in fact battle plan methods to deal with the sane in part. Adica cum timpita e sanatos la cap.

The sane publish battle plans that are to be used to destroy them. This is why Jesus calls them the dead because everything goes right over their head, everything. Perhaps I should not have mentioned that but on second thought the sane cannot understand anything I say ever. In contrast to how the ecological system was around the time written language was invented about 5400 to 7000 years ago until right now, essentially the ecological systems have all been destroyed. So the sane perceive they have a right to destroy an ecological system because the laws created by the sane suggest they can. Taigi vienintelis tikrasis tirpalas yra Raudonoji jūra sprendimus, ir kad yra skirtumas tarp šių kairėje smegenų obrzydliwości ir tie, kurie yra sveiko proto, stengiasi išlaikyti juos sunaikinti viską, kas konflikto. The conflict is what is known as good versus evil. The wise ones, who can live in harmony with the surroundings, and the beast's who destroy everything in their path, including their own first born.

[Genesis 11:5 And the LORD came down to see the city and the tower, which the children of men builded.]
Even today the sane build towers to heaven as if these material towers will improve their minds somehow. The sane will argue they need the towers in order to conserve space but the whole reason they are running out of space is because they have unsound minds and overpopulate the entire planet. The sane create the problems and then do things that only create more problems. Abraham knew if he burned their towers they would panic because the sane are no longer capable of living off the land because they only have left brain sequential intelligence to support them. One might suggest the wise brought down the vain towers of the worshipers of the whore demotic. History has saepenumero ipsum.
Abraham was very wise although the sane will never grasp how wise Abraham really was. Civilization itself is a symptom of beings that have been conditioned into an unsound state of mind, extreme left brain state, caused by the written education and so civilization itself is doomed to fall apart at the seams because it was built by minds that are unsound and thus like the sand. There is no indication of harmony in civilization only conflicts that rely on conflicts to exist.

9/5/2009 4:30:28 AM –

[Genesis 11:8 So the LORD scattered them abroad from thence upon the face of all the earth: and they left off to build the city.

Gen 11:9 Therefore is the name of it called Babel; because the LORD did there confound the language of all the earth: and from thence did the LORD scatter them abroad upon the face of all the earth.]

This denotes written language created many different versions of the written language and it separated people and thus created nations of people who knew these select languages. They all went their own way to build their cities. So the cities are not a symptom of progress they are a symptom of the written language. The written language changed people's minds and one of the side effects is people started acting differently and started building cities. So the cities are called Babel in relation to the ones who are of unsound mind. There are various written languages and they separate people so one group Babbles or cannot be understood by another group. So this created labels. So today we have one country that does not speak the language of another country so they perceive they are different when in reality they are not different. They had to separate because for example one could not have a city where there were 20 languages spoken or 20 dominate languages. It would be far too confusing so these groups have to separate and create their own cities of just people who spoke one language.

[Genesis 13:2 And Abram was very rich in cattle, in silver, and in gold.

Genesis 13:5 And Lot also, which went with Abram, had flocks, and herds, and tents.]

The thing that makes these texts so complex is the sane only see parts so they assume every time a word is used it means the same thing. The ones who are awake only see things as a whole so they may have many different ways to say for example cattle. So the comments suggest Abram was rich in cattle. The sane will assume

Abram had actual cattle but in this case cattle is a way of saying ones he assisted using the covenant, fear not.

[Genesis 12:5 And Abram took Sarai his wife, and Lot his brother's son, and all their substance that they had gathered, and the souls that they had gotten in Haran; and they went forth to go into the land of Canaan; and into the land of Canaan they came.]

"The souls they had gotten in Haran" denotes the ones they told the fear not remedy to and then in a later comment it says Abram was rich with cattle and so cattle and souls mean the same thing. Silver and gold in the comment denotes cerebral wealth. So these comments are relative to this comment.

[Genesis 15:1 After these things the word of the LORD came unto Abram in a vision, saying, Fear not, Abram: I am thy shield, and thy exceeding great reward.]
So Abram "woke up" and discovered the fear not remedy so he had exceeding great reward or vast cerebral riches and so these riches were also many cattle or souls or ones he assisted with the fear not remedy. They were not his slaves they were simply ones he assisted to the "promise land" or to mental sound mind. So Abraham was a wise man because he understood the key or remedy to the written language which was fear not.

[Genesis 13:5 And Lot also, which went with Abram, had flocks, and herds, and tents.]
This comment suggest Lot was also a wise man like Abram and understood the remedy fear not. "Had flocks" denotes Lot had many he assisted with the remedy. Tent's denotes they were hunters and gatherers much like Native Americans were. This is in contrast to the ones in the cities who had houses and thus were fixed in their locations. Simply put Abram and Lot were in tribes not in civilization or cities.

This fear not remedy is spoken so it is words and words are sounds and sounds are intangible. One cannot catch a sound in a bottle so to speak. Applying the fear not remedy is a mental or mind aspect and mind is also intangible. So one hears the words fear not and applies that remedy to the curse which is mental conditioning away from fear, so in one respect nothing happens or nothing tangible happens, but in another respect one's mind changes and everything they think and sense after the remedy is applied changes or ones whole mental perception changes. So the paradox to the fear not remedy is nothing happens and everything happens. Perhaps that needs some clarification. I will talk about myself since I have an infinite ego and I understand the alternative.

I was sick from taking the pills and I thought I need to get help and then I thought I won't seek help. That was a mental decision and is not tangible on the scale of physical measurements yet everything I have written in these diaries since that time are a result of that decision. So what really happened in that room that night was nothing. It was a split second mental decision that is not tangible. It is not measurable or it is beyond the realms of measurement. So that is the paradox, one could suggest nothing happened and one could also argue much happened. Perhaps all that happened in that room was mental self control and that is intangible. One may see the fruits or symptoms of that self control event but one can never capture that mental self control decision and measure it.

[Luke 17:33 … and whosoever shall lose his life shall preserve it.]

Once a person applies the above mental self control suggestion properly everything changes for them mentally yet it is immeasurable or unnamable as to exactly what happens. Perhaps suggesting one increases their mental heightened awareness is as good as any description. To clarify. A veces yo pierdo atraso.

The center of happiness is you and if you don't buy that then it's me. My only problem with morals is people expect me to live by the ones I suggest I have.

[Genesis 13:6 And the land was not able to bear them, that they might dwell together: for their substance was great, so that they could not dwell together.]

This is what overpopulation does to our species. The land or ecological system cannot bear the sane because the sane have way to many offspring because they do not have the mental ability to understand what is going to happen if they keep destroying everything in their path and having children like rabbits with no thought to the consequences.

If I had morals I wouldn't be talking to you would I. Common sense is a misunderstanding the majority is not aware of. If common sense was common we would all be happy. Winning is a luxury we all afford to fail at. Failing costs very little and helps one understand winning.

I was in a chat room and I typed a sentence and misspelled a word. A person in that chat room said "Whatever you are saying it cannot be right because you cannot even spell." It occurred to me they were mimicking their teachers in school. On one level; they boost their self up by pointing out they can see a misspelled word, so they are insulting the person who misspelled the word and in turn they get satisfaction knowing they would have never misspelled that word. This is a type of mental gratification but it is based on the fallacy that if a person misspells a word they are stupid and that is what a teacher induces in students.

A teacher looks at the spelling test and determines who is stupid and who is wise by who spells all the words properly. So here these people in the chat rooms many years after they were taught written language and they are mimicking what their teacher taught them: If one does not spell a word properly they are not intelligent. So these people are grading me on my spelling yet I do not pay them to grade me and so they are charitable. They do not have to grade me on my spelling but they take time out of their day to let me know when I misspell a word so they charitable and they are slaves to the written language.

Every time I misspell a word they take time out of their busy life to grade me. These people cannot stand when they see a misspelled word. Scientists have shown the word does not need to be spelled properly for the brain to determine what the word is. Right brain is very good at patterns and can easily fill in the blanks or letters that are out of sequence yet the people in extreme left brain cannot let a misspelled word stand without grading the person who misspells the word. I understand on some mental level every person is aware of what this written language education has done to them mentally and many go out of their way to make sure it does the same to everyone. It's cerebral so perhaps I am not explaining it properly.

They scold me for not spelling a word right and so they perceive that will make me fall in line and spell that word right next time. They have become minions of the demotic script. They police it and make sure everyone spells properly but they do it on the guise that they are wise because they can spell words properly. Their entire standard of wisdom is that they can put letters in the proper sequence according to the rules of the language. To them wisdom is being a good mimic. Relative to their understanding anyone who does not follow the spelling rules is not intelligent or wise and in fact stupid. So their gauge of wisdom and intelligence is not even logical or sane.

A word processor never spells a word wrong because it has the word in its memory but that does not mean it is intelligent it only means it's a good mimic. So these people correct my spelling and they perceive it is because they are wise and teaching me but in reality I only understand they are some sort of judge that basis their understanding on flawed logic. I understand they perceive I am there to spell the words properly so they will accept me but in truth I do not care if the words are spelled properly because I am aware they know I am saying anyway. They spell these words properly their whole life and they are waiting for wisdom to kick in. They got the education so why are they not great thinkers, or great inventors, or great wise ones? When does this great wisdom from learning written language kick in? When do they get smart? I do not detect smart. I detect mimics emulating their teachers attempting to persuade me their spelling proves they have brain function. I feel sad for them and I pray for ignorance. I will end on that note before I implode. - 1:12:41 PM

1:28:28 PM – So 5400 years ago a person invented written language and brought in ten students to teach it to. Three of the students picked up on it and started to spell words in proper sequence and the remaining seven did not and so they were send out to build the pyramids and become slaves. So this inventor of the written language made a judgment call based on the premise if one cannot learn his invention they are stupid. That is a false premise because the species lived for perhaps 200,000 years without written language at all. So then there is big problem now.

The written language invention as well as math threw us into extreme left brain and thus altered how we act. We now over populate. We now kill off all other species. We now kill ourselves as in suicide. We now kill each other for money and land as opposed to just for self defense. So nature is taking care of the mistake. So nature is a delicate balance and any species that gets out of balance cannot last. So as we look at the world what is happening is we are really looking at our species killing itself off, because this invention threw our minds out of balance and so we are dying off by killing our life sustaining environment and our minds are so unbalanced we cannot even tell that is what we are doing or what is happening.

I am not suggesting some supernatural aspect is going to come and kill us. I am suggesting we as a species, because we push this left brain conditioning on everyone, are now so mentally unbalanced we are killing ourselves off and we as a species do not have the mental capacity to understand that is what is happening. I do not detect anything supernatural here. I detect a species that inadvertently altered its mind and is no longer viable. Nature is taking care of the mistake so to speak. The dinosaurs lived for well over 100 million years.

The sane cannot think clearly so they perceive everything is just fine. They attempt to think but cannot think. They attempt to suggest six billion people is viable or possible in relation to survival. I am aware it is too late. That is all I know. I will not suggest it can be turned around because that's a lie. All I see is a 5000 year old mistake that is now catching up to us. Perhaps the sane can tell it's starting to show.

We as a species are of unsound mind and so we perceive we are above everything else and so everything else is expendable. That is because as a species we are so unsound in mind because of the demotic invention we cannot tell what reality is. The sane will go around and suggest supernatural aspects will correct everything but that is because they are no longer able to think so they rest on supernatural aspect saving them in the end.

The sane perceive supernatural aspects will trump nature. They are simply so mentally unsound they no longer can tell what reality is. I do not care we are killing ourselves off as a species because this invention has made us mentally unsound and thus unviable. I do not care because it is far too late to change anything. All I detect is the sane running around suggesting they can make more money if they destroy more forests and build a few houses and to hell with the creatures that live there. That is all that has happened for the last 5000 years or more in relation to the sane. This unsound mind as a result of the education has given the sane this mental god complex.

The sane perceive they are greater than nature itself even though they are in reality not even relevant to nature itself. Nature does not care about our species at all. Nature creates and kills million of species and never blinks. Somehow this extreme left brain state we have conditioned ourselves into makes us think we are greater than what enabled us to exist in the first place. In reality we are a delicate species. Vast population does not mean we are not delicate it means we are mentally unsound because we would not have such a huge population if we were mentally sound.

I am not preaching. I am not one who perceives I can reverse a 5000 year old mistake. The sane are still building houses as if the earth is infinite in size. The sane are unable to grasp there is no other planet within light years of earth that can sustain us. The sane kill everything for a dollar because someone told them if they get the education and make money they are wise.

In reality a brain dead mole cricket has infinite wisdom in contrast to the sane because a brain dead mole cricket does not kill the grass that sustains it. We went from a mammal that lived in harmony with nature for 200,000 years and then we made this invention and it altered our minds way too far to the left and now we are suicidal as a species. I understand that is nature's solution to this mistake.

The species is suicidal so the species as a whole is of unsound mind. I saw a show were a biologist found some tiger fish off the coast of Florida and he said "We need to kill them off when we find them because they will mess up the ecological system here."

I understand a brain dead mole cricket does not describe the sane properly. This biologist has a god complex because he assumes our species can never do anything wrong and any other species can only do things wrong. The sane eat three meals a day and are still hungry after that so all I can assume is they are gluttonous pigs.

The sane hog everything. Everything in the path of the sane is destroyed. Not some things, not most things, but everything. I tend to fall back on my previous assumption that I in fact did die in that last suicide attempt and I am in hell. Then I realize the world was the same as it is now before that last attempt so then I consider the reason I wanted to die is because I am in hell and then I realize I cannot escape hell if I am in hell. I jump back up on the fence because I need to experiment more and if it is hell that's all one can do is experiment and if it is not hell perhaps it is the hell of hell.

Perhaps it is the hell the ones in hell go to when they are too dammed for hell itself. I look at hell as being aware of a problem but being unable to do anything about it. Hell is the inability to change the evitable. Hell is the inability to communicate reason. Hell is the inability to detect hell when one is in it. Maybe you should tell yourself everything is going to be just fine so it will not hurt as much. I do not feel anything so I am pleased with the reality. If this section was on topic, call. I need all the filler I can get.- 2:13:18 PM

Being right or being wrong is not as important as being.

2:42:38 PM – I try to stay in the realm of left brain right brain so now I will go to a supernatural perspective and then jump back on the fence. This whole fear not concept in relation to the Abraham and Isaac story and this comment among others may mean one thing. [Luke 17:33 … and whosoever shall lose his life shall preserve it.]

One faces perceived death and then allows it and so the mind is tricked into dying but the body remains alive. So this would mean this method fear not may just be a way to mentally die and enjoy the rewards of afterlife yet still be physically alive. One has slight emotions and slight hunger and has extreme concentration so life becomes very easy .Sense of time is reduced so life also becomes very long.

So perhaps this concept of defeating death means you mentally are in the afterlife but physically still alive so you defeat death because you mentally die but are still alive physically. So one mentally loses their life and they preserve their body because they are no longer nervous because emotions are turned down. They do not eat so much so they do not have as much wear and tear on the body. They do not get upset and stressed for long periods so they live longer.

This take would mean humans found a way to trick their mind into thinking it died and then it would start acting like it died, yet the person would remain physically alive and so then they started telling people this discovery. There are many people who have near death experiences and then suggest their outlook changed.

I understand there is a difference between someone who has a near death experience as a result of an accident or illness and someone who is suicidal and seeking death yet does not pull it off but accomplishes the "waking up". No matter what this fear not technique does it is still in the realm of psychology or at least parapsychology. So I do not detect supernatural because I am supernatural so I am not afraid of myself, and ones who fear supernatural are not aware they are supernatural so they still afraid of their self. This would mean written language made us left brained and thus afraid and made us blind to what we are. I assure you I can jump back on the fence much faster than you can. - 3:02:40 PM

9/6/2009 6:07:57 AM

[Genesis 13:6 And the land was not able to bear them, that they might dwell together: for their substance was great, so that they could not dwell together.

7 And there was a strife between the herdmen of Abram's cattle and the herdmen of Lot's cattle: and the Canaanite and the Perizzite dwelled then in the land.

8 And Abram said unto Lot, Let there be no strife, I pray thee, between me and thee, and between my herdmen and thy herdmen; for we be brethren.]

This comment is not what it appears to be. These tribes did not have herds of cattle they were wanders or nomads or hunters and gatherers. So the cattle comment refers to

[Genisis 3:14 "thou art cursed above all cattle".]

The cattle were the ones who they were trying to assist. The herdsmen were similar to their assistants. This is typical for ones who wake up. They are lone wolves. That is kind of why the ones who wake up, team never wins, because they do not work in groups.

The sane work well in groups because they cannot think for their self so they perceive there is power in numbers. The ones who are awake prefer solitary efforts. One example is look at the disciples. They all went their separate ways to suggest the fear not remedy. This can be applied to modern day.

Edison and Tesla tried to work together but it never really panned out. Einstein also liked to work alone. So the end of this passage is saying "for we are brethren" which means we are both awake, Lot and Abraham, but they split up. When one is awake they cannot actually hold a grudge or be angry so they were not angry they just prefer to be lone wolves or go it alone. So this comment is showing Lot and Abraham were the wise ones or the ones fully awake and their herdsman were getting close to being fully awake and then they had the cattle which were ones who needed assistance to become awake, or who were still under the fear curse. It would be real nice to just be able to say to someone fear not and then they would go apply it but the reality is their fear is so great it will not allow them to apply [Luke 17:33 … and whosoever shall lose his life shall preserve it.]. They must be led to the water strategically and I don't have patience for that because I have infinite books to write.

None of the sane are going to apply this remedy without lots of fighting and arguments because they perceive how they are mentally is perfectly normal, when in fact they are perfectly mentally abnormal. They got twelve years of left brain conditioning, it is impossible they are mentally sound but they do not understand that. They perceive all the fear they have is totally natural. It is not really like Abraham and Lot were trying to wake all these people, that is not exactly how it works. They were just going about doing what they do and these people were interested in what they suggested because they were wise.

The sane are curious about wise beings but the wise being use that to suggest things that may lead the sane to the "promise land" so to speak, which is consciousness. So the comment cattle in the above comments refers to this comment about cattle earlier in the Chapter.

[Genesis 3:14 …..And the LORD God said unto the serpent, Because thou hast done this, thou art cursed above all cattle,…]

And interesting note here is, the ones who got the education are considered the serpent or exhibit mental symptoms of what is known as the seven deadly sins and that is why they are cursed above cattle. Their mental state is the seven deadly sins so that means they are the serpent and so they are mentally cursed if they do not apply the remedy, fear not. So they get the education and become cursed and do not apply the remedy and then they teach it their children and curse their children, even their first born, and so the curse just spreads, so the cursed beget curses and that is also a part of the curse. The cursed create more cursed. It's a self sustaining curse. - 6:37:07 AM

I am not ashamed to suggest in contrast to how I mentally was for forty years I am now mentally alive. I am not ashamed to say I was certainly mentally cursed in contrast to how I am mentally

39

now just ten months since the accident. This world cannot change that ever. I do not fear this world because I understand the cursed, because I was cursed.

I do not care if the world suggests I am arrogant for saying that because the world in fact cursed me so to begin with their attempts to making me wise with education. The world is so cursed it attempts to makes wise beings wise with its education and only makes wise beings cursed, so the world of the sane means less than nothing to me.

They perceive many of the diseases they deal with are symptoms of nature when in reality they are symptoms of the curse. The sane try to make it sound like they are proud of their diseases. They brought the diseases with them and then suggest the American Indians were savages because the Indians did not have the diseases they had. The reality is the diseases they brought were because of the curse and then they cursed the Indians.

The diseases are because of the cities. The Black death plague is a good example. The fact of the cities is a reason for the plague. This is all relative to the curse. The curse denotes everything is cursed and anything one who is under the curse touches becomes cursed. The sane curse everything and that is the nature of a curse. Once one breaks the curse by applying fear not they are immune to ones who are cursed. One is able to live among the cursed but not become cursed again because they have broken the curse.

[Hebrews 6:4 For it is impossible for those who were once enlightened, and have tasted of the heavenly gift, and were made partakers of the Holy Ghost,]

Long story short, once one applies the remedy and becomes enlightened, unveils right brain, they cannot be cursed again. One becomes an observer of the cursed and there are around six billion to observe. One might suggest the cursed are like the grains of sand in the sea. - 7:17:14 AM

We tried to fly away but kept landing back here.

So we clipped our wings in hopes we would eventually forget we ever could fly.

I soon forgot about the sky and forgot about the high.

I soon forgot to even try; the only way to reject their lie.

The viper has many heads thus my sword of ink is very sharp.

Illic es plures mores neco a viper tamen plurrimi efficens ratio est ut discerpo suus caput capitis.

A skilled hunter can convince a viper to bite itself.

2:23:52 PM – The oldest known city Hamoukar is in Syria. It is understood this city was around roughly 4000 BC which means it is about 6000 years old. Written language was invented around that time perhaps 5400 years ago and maybe even up to 7000 years ago. The point being there will never be a city found that predates written language because written language altered human beings minds and that is what created the cities or made man decide to build cities.

Man needed the cities because he left the wilderness. The language altered mans mind so far to the left they became something they are not. They needed cities and shelters all the sudden. They need to build towers to heaven all of the sudden. They lived in the wilderness just fine for 200,000 years and then they needed to build towers to heaven all the sudden.

[Gen 11:5 And the LORD came down to see the city and the tower, which the children of men builded.]

It is such an obvious connection yet the sane will never ever figure it out. Their minds cannot grasp the obvious. Man invented language and math and then started building cities. Is it because we got smarter or because we became mentally unsound? Either mankind got smarter or mankind got dumber but there is no other option.

[Genesis 3:6 And when the woman saw that the tree was good for food, and that it was pleasant to the eyes, and a tree to be desired to make one wise, she took of the fruit thereof, and did eat, and gave also unto her husband with her; and he did eat.]

Of course written language looked good for the mind. Of course written language looks pleasing to the eyes with it's pretty characters and all written languages are pretty to look at. Of course written language makes one wise. We are certainly wise now aren't we? You have destroyed everything with your assumptions of wisdom. - 2:36:31 PM

5:40:11 PM – The true tragedy with the left brain education is it conditions a person to hate right brain. There are two hemispheres of the brain for a reason. These two hemispheres are contrary. This means they are opposite and totally opposite. Written language is based on sequence as in the ABC's are in sequence and the spelling of words are in sequence as well as the structure of sentences for example getting the tenses of the sentence in proper sequence. This is all left brain characteristics and thus all left brain conditioning.

Then one of these people experiences a person who has right brain unveiled and they see them as babbling but that babbling is really random access thoughts. So it's not babbling it's really that left brain conditioned person is experiencing was a sound minded person is like. When a person or teacher scolds someone for not spelling a word properly they are really saying they hate right brain. They are conditioned so far to the left they hate the complex random access aspect of their mind. They are mentally a house divided and thus mentally they cannot stand. They cannot mentally function because their complex random access powerhouse is veiled to such an extreme they actually need to take drugs to even feel it.

This is perhaps the worst part of the curse. The curse makes a person hate their own mind. They may insult me for misspelling words or not being able to stay on topic but in reality they are saying they hate half of their brain. They are saying they hate the complex aspect of their mind. They hate the creative, complex, random access aspect of their thoughts. They do not hate me. They have been conditioned to hate their mind. I do not detect any supernatural entity would do this to us. I detect we invented something that looked very pleasing and seemed too good to be true and it certainly was too good to be true. I understand we could do this to ourselves. I do not detect any entity that could be as wicked to us as we are to ourselves. We made life very hard on ourselves mentally with this invention written language and that's the harshest truth of all. I understand the enemy and I cannot convince him we are old friends.- 5:48:47 PM

8:25:00 PM – One great misunderstanding is that material things are bad. Material things are inanimate. Cities are simply buildings and they are inanimate. Technology is inanimate. It's not possible these things can be bad. Many of the suggestions about the cities and the towers built to heaven were relative to characteristics the ones who got the education and did not apply the remedy were showing.

Right brain is the creative aspect of the mind. Creativity is relative to adaptation. So when the right brain is veiled a person does not like change because they are unable to adapt to it easily and then they end up in stagnation. The sane tend to get stuck in a rut as it were. They find a set pattern of living and they stick to it their whole life. They do not like change. Contrast that to the American Indians, they were able to break camp and move to a new location at the spur of the moment. Contrast that to early man who was a hunter and gatherer. Early man wandered in the wilderness and adapted to anything that came along. So when the right brain is veiled the creativity is silenced and so is the adaptation ability so then life becomes much harder than it has to be or than it should be. - 8:32:27 PM

10:48:30 PM – Genesis explains everything one ever needs to know and it does it in the first 15 chapters. Everything beyond the first 15 chapters is simply details reinforcing the principle spirit of the first 15 chapters. This includes all ancient religious texts. It is no more complex than that.

First there is the problem. There is a problem that happened or occurred. The characteristics of this problem are explained.

[Genesis 3:6 And when the woman saw that the tree was good for food, and that it was pleasant to the eyes, and a tree to be desired to make one wise, she took of the fruit thereof, and did eat, and gave also unto her husband with her; and he did eat.]

So the characteristics of the problem looked good for food or knowledge , was pleasing to the eyes to look at and it was assumed it made one wise or intelligent to "eat" this food.

So the problem is written language. That is the only thing at this period of time in history it could be because it was relatively new.

The next part is what this problem causes or does.

[Genesis 3:10 And he said, I heard thy voice in the garden, and I was afraid, because I was naked; and I hid myself.]

It makes one mentally afraid and this comment suggest it makes one mentally ashamed which could also be described as shy and that is a symptom of an unsound mind.

[Genesis 2:25 And they were both naked, the man and his wife, and were not ashamed.]

So simply put before they learned written language they were not afraid and not ashamed and after the tree of knowledge they were ashamed and were afraid. So this suggests a mental perception change. So that means their mental state changed. Clinically they went extreme left brain from learning a strictly sequential based invention.

So now we have the problem, written language and the symptoms one exhibits after they learn written language, fear and shame among other things.

Then there is the remedy in chapter 15.

[Genesis 15:1 After these things the word of the LORD came unto Abram in a vision, saying, Fear not, Abram: I am thy shield, and thy exceeding great reward.]

The fear conditioning is what negates the left brain conditioning and one return's to sound mind they get to keep language and nothing else is required after that. The fear conditioning is a onetime thing, that is what repent means, simply apply the fear conditioning and return to sound mind. So in reality there is no point in religion at all.

Once one applies the remedy and that takes one night if one wants the fast route and then everything else takes care of itself. The whole principle of confession and ask for forgiveness and pray for salvation, that is all just some money making scheme. No deity is going to make you condition away the fear you have to do it yourself and use your mind.

I am not compelled to pray or mediate. I am not compelled to ask anything of anyone. I am not ashamed. I am not afraid. I do not need to pray. I was meek for one second because I let go when my left brain wanted me to call for help. I do not need to worry about being meek ever again. Meek is a onetime thing just like repent. If you do it properly one time is enough for both. I am done with trying to get better. I am in a situation if I pray I will be praying for ignorance not wisdom. I do not want to know anymore. Simply put I know far more than I wanted to know.

If you are still praying then you have no applied fear not properly. If you have applied fear not properly you are in neutral mentally. That means you do not have anything to ask for. What I am saying is organized religion is a money making opportunity and has nothing to do with the ancient texts. One is either going to apply the remedy, fear not, or they are not. There is nothing to discuss. There is nothing to pray about. There is nothing to debate. There is nothing to give money for. One either applies the remedy or they do not and that is up to them.

There is no need to charge people money for telling them this remedy unless one is only in it for the money. You will not find me having a seminar or a speaking engagement because it has nothing to do with me. I already applied the remedy accidentally. I have nothing to say to anyone. They can read and they can understand the remedy and its all on their shoulders not my shoulders. I certainly could turn this into a new religion but I do not give a dam about money so I won't be turning this in to a new religion.

No one is going to be turning my name into a money making opportunity or a holiday or any of that crap. I do not want anyone to idolize me. I prefer they idolize their self and rely on their own mind and not try to make it seem like I am special because I suggest they are exactly like me they just perhaps need to work on that log of fear in their mind a bit.

I fail if anyone concludes I am gifted or special or tapped. Everyone has a brain and some minds have varying degrees of fear and the equation is, the less fear they have in their mind the better. Every time a person defeats a fear they increase the right brain and the greatest fear of all is fear of perceived death so if one just cuts to the chase and defeats that fear all the others fears are taken care of. That is what these texts are all about.

[Genesis 15:1 After these things the word of the LORD came unto Abram in a vision, saying, Fear not, Abram: I am thy shield, and thy exceeding great reward.]

You get the fear out and you get an exceedingly great reward and you can do it in one night so it is not a lifelong profession. There is no reason build a shrine for it or charge people money for it unless one is in it for the money. It would be nice if money could get that fear out of your head but that is not the case and it never will be. - 11:32:07 PM

9/7/2009 7:29:06 PM – These two comments are related.

[Genesis 15:1 After these things the word of the LORD came unto Abram in a vision, saying, Fear not, Abram: I am thy shield, and thy exceeding great reward.]

[Genesis 21:17 And God heard the voice of the lad; and the angel of God called to Hagar out of heaven, and said unto her, What aileth thee, Hagar? fear not; for God hath heard the voice of the lad where he is.]

Hagar was a female and Egyptian. Egyptian is code word for one who was in civilization or taught the written language and has not applied the remedy. Moses was in civilization also before he broke the curse. So these comments keep referring to Egypt but that is because at this time and place Egypt was pushing the written language. Egypt had variations of Hieroglyphics.

They had the fancy form which was used in the pyramids and they also had everyday script or demotic. It is similar to a person knowing how to write and another person being able to write using very fancy penmanship. "What aileth thee Hagar" denotes Hagar had the curse. Then the remedy is suggested, fear not.

What this means is this book of Genesis is attempting to show various people who woke up from the extreme left brain demotic induced mental state and then they explain how they did. This is not suggesting these were the first people to wake up from the neurosis because written language was around much longer than 2500 BC. Genesis is simply the first written text found that explained the curse and then the testaments of people who broke the curse. So it is saying this written language, tree of knowledge, messed our minds up and this is how we broke that curse.

So all of these people who are understood to be on the side of "god" are simply people who got the education and then broke the mental curse it caused. Theses wise beings are trying to make a case. They are trying to convince the ones who are still cursed they have witnesses that it is a curse. Of course they failed and the sane never got the message and the proof is the entire world is still educating

47

the kids with the written language and never suggest the remedy which is fear not or fear conditioning. Simply put one perhaps cannot break the curse any other way but with fear conditioning and even then it takes a time for the mind to get back into proper form.

It is like one who is in a deep sleep and then they wake up and they are cranky and irritable. So all of these wise beings throughout the world who broke this curse in one way or another failed with their texts. They all failed. The sane never got the point because one cannot convince a blind man blindness is abnormal. This is all a symptom of how devastating the written language is in relation to what it does to a person's mind.

Moses only attacked the sane after he exhausted all his words. Moses realized he could not prove to the sane they were mentally unsound with words and he also could not do it with war. This denotes this neurosis is so far out of control is it completely hopeless in relation to the species. All one needs to think about is, human beings lived for perhaps 200,000 years in harmony with nature and in the wilderness and in 5000 years or so we have this ecological nightmare and overpopulation and inability to feed everyone and depression and suicides and vast wars that never seem to end.

There is only thing that caused all of that and it is because human beings are conditioned in extreme left brain under the guise of education. It is not even important if anyone believes that because they cannot stop it and none of these wise being from thousands of years ago could stop it. This is because the written language induced neurosis is fatal to the species. Human beings literally killed their self with the invention that seemed pleasing to the eyes and seemed like it would make them wise.

[Genesis 3:6 And when the woman saw that the tree was good for food, and that it was pleasant to the eyes, and a tree to be desired to make one wise, she took of the fruit thereof, and did eat, and gave also unto her husband with her; and he did eat.]

When a person is a child and they start getting this left brain indoctrination their mind is not even fully developed so by the time their mind is fully developed they have perhaps 8 to 10 years of this left brain education so they cannot even tell what has happened to their mind. The "experts" also had this happen to their mind so they are mentally damaged to. The doctors had this happen to them so they are mentally damaged to. Everyone got this left brain education so they are all mentally damaged so they cannot help anyone because they cannot even tell they are mentally damaged. Only a person who has a near death experience and in fact seeks to die, which is one who is suicidal, can fully wake up and it is accidental.

[Luke 17:33 ; and whosoever shall lose his life shall preserve it.]

This comment is a suicidal person. In Buddhism it is suggested one be mindful of death. If you go into a psychologist and say you are mindful of death they will prescribe you anti-depressants. The bottom line to this situation is of course once one gets the education it is perhaps impossible to wake up intentionally. I speak to ones who are working their way to waking up and some spend their whole life doing it and never quite wake up fully, or what is known as go the full measure. If one goes to the Amazon and finds those tribes who live in the Amazon they are the last vestiges of human beings of sound mind.

Once one gets the education their mind is damaged goods. They can wake up and negate the extreme left brain conditioning but their mind is still damaged. It's simply mental damage that can ever be fully undone. The sane cannot ever grasp that because their whole world would shatter if they for one second understand that was absolute fact. The complexity is these wise beings thousands of years ago tried to warn us and the sane never ever got it. One might argue they didn't have the proper way to explain it but the truth is I can explain it strictly psychologically but the sane cannot admit they are perhaps damaged goods.

Some psychologist can relate to what I say and also some who understand the brain but I am uncertain if they would ever attempt the fear conditioning because after all it is mental suicide. I understand the depressed are very aware something is wrong. They want to get the hell out of here, simply put. The ones who run around and babble about how wonderful everything is, they are clueless beyond the realms of understanding. So they are so far into neurosis they see a nightmare as daylight. No words are going to solve this situation and no war is going to solve this situation which means there is no solution to this situation. That's the only truth I understand. In case you think it is just me here is a comment from one I spoke with in a chat room and they are in agreement.

[23:04] <EmilyE> Yeah, exactly. You really can't teach anyone.

[23:08] <EmilyE> I just see it as pointless really. Help people as you can, make things better for each other, because we're all one, ya know?

This is what this concept of everything is pointless is all about. This being has given up the fight because they have the powerhouse right brain unveiled and they can see it is pointless in short order. The sane generally only have sequential thoughts which is left brain, are quite slothful mentally in coming to conclusions so it has taken them 2500 years to try to figure out elementary ancient texts about this "curse" and they still haven't figured it out, and now it's far too late. Everyone is going down in the sinking ship. I don't have emotions so I am indifferent. How do you feel about it? Perhaps you should pray I am wrong. The critical mass has passed and we are in the implosion stage. The sane just keep ruining the next generations mind with the education and then do not even bother to apply the fear not remedy so every single thing the sane do is meaningless because the root cause of all the problems is never ever addressed. One might suggest the logic of the sane is infinitely slightly unsound. I agree with all of these wise beings from the past but that does not mean I agree with you.- 8:12:17 PM

8:20:46 AM – [Genesis 17:5 Neither shall thy name any more be called Abram, but thy name shall be Abraham; for a father of many nations have I made thee.

Genesis 17:6 And I will make thee exceeding fruitful, and I will make nations of thee, and kings shall come out of thee.]

This is where Abram changed his name to Abraham. The father of many nations is suggesting Abraham holds the key or covenant which is the remedy fear not. So the father of many nations means Abraham will be able to assist people to break the curse using his patented Abraham and Isaac technique which is what fear not is. This is relative to the comment a house divided among itself cannot stand.

So when one is extreme left brained they have an unsound mind and thus fear and then Abraham suggests the fear not remedy and then a person goes back to sound mind and they are whole again. So Abraham creates many "nations" or brings people out of the curse. So the exceedingly fruitful means Abraham can assist many to break the curse. "Kings shall come out of thee" denotes he will assist many to become kings of the house/mind. So when one applies this remedy Abraham suggests they return to sounds mind and become kings again and return from the dead, mentally speaking.

Granted this is all water under the bridge because Abraham didn't convince enough people. Abraham didn't try hard enough. Abraham failed as bad as one could ever fail because he was dealing with mentally damaged goods that would not understand truth if it was speaking to them. Is est quare EGO operor non effigies ullus illorum sapiens res quoniam they deficio nos. Forsitan they should have exuro down pauci magis civis. Si they erant dignitas suum sal salis nos wouldn't exsisto fatum iam would nos? Si EGO reputo quisquam illorum sapiens res EGO reputo they erant non incidere sicco pro officium. In reality written language was spread throughout the world so there was no way to stop the curse.

The deeper meaning in this comment is proof this is not a supernatural situation. If this was a supernatural situation and not a psychological situation all these wise beings would not have failed so miserably. All these wise beings failed miserably because they could not reach the beings who were extreme left brained. I do not detect a lick of supernatural. I detect beings in full neurosis that are unable to understand beings that are of sound mind.

I submit some people understand what I suggest but when it comes right down to it they are not going to apply fear not or pull an Abraham and Isaac. They are not going to lose their self to preserve it. This is because they are fear based and Abraham and Isaac technique requires one to ignore fear so the sane will never do that. It is all really a joke because it's simply too late. This left brain indoctrination is incurable. Since is it incurable the species mentally is unsound and so nature is going to make sure the species kills itself off because nature does not allow unviable species to survive.

This is the situation. There is a bubble and that is earth and nature is outside of that bubble and nature see's this unsound unviable creature in the bubble and it is exhibiting fruits that just destroy everything around it so this creature that is unviable no longer lives in harmony with the other creatures in the bubble. So nature separates the good creatures or the wheat from the bad creature the chaff. Nature will allow that unviable mentally unsound creature to destroy itself because nature does not allow mutations to survive because mutations are not able to live in harmony with the entire ecological system.

So man has all these problems that are showing up in the bubble or earth and man cannot solve them. Is mankind living in harmony with the environment or is mankind this run away dominate above all other things creature? The tricky part is one of unsound mind cannot answer that question because they do not have the mental capacity to fully grasp the situation. That is what the curse is really all about.

The ones conditioned all the way to the left cannot see the reality, they cannot think clearly. They cannot find solutions and so they simply talk their self into some alternative reality. They try to explain all of these symptoms away using reason that is not even reality. The problems are so deep or so complex the sane cannot mentally grasp them. The sane see depression as just a normal part of life. The sane see building cities and tearing down all the ecological systems as a normal part of life. The sane see the children harming their self with drugs and killing their self and suggest that is a normal part of life. The sane see people over eating and dying from all of the addictions and suggest that is a normal part of life. The sane cannot grasp what is really happening is these mentally unsound creatures are killing their self off because that's the way nature deals with unsound unviable creatures.

Some of the sane will suggest what I suggest is truth and they agree with it but they do not. They get it half way. They agree with some things but they never can get to the bottom line. The bottom line is the written education man keeps throwing on the next generation dooms the next generation and it keeps dooming every generation. This is not about aliens or ghost or any crap like that, this is about taking a sound minded child and conditioning them so far to the left and then not applying the remedy, they in fact simply create unviable creatures that cannot function in an ecological system.

What I suggest is absolute fact but absolute fact is far beyond the mental capabilities of the sane. The sane will suggest technology will save them but technology cannot compete with a mentally unviable creature because nature will not allow a mentally unviable creature. Nature kills off mutations. It is no more complex than that. All the problems in society are simply proof nature is making us kill our self off because nature does not like mutations in its harmonious ecological system.

There are many examples of creatures that simply did not cut the mustard and were in turn killed off in one way or another naturally. So mankind invented written language and it inadvertently altered our minds and made us unsound in mind and then we lost our ability to live in harmony with the ecological and now it is showing, that mentally speaking as a species we are unviable. One could just take a group of gorillas and cut out their right brain and let them loose in nature and one would see they would die off swiftly because they could not function in any kind of lasting way.

So this is not about human beings being genetically mutated, this is about human beings making an invention that inadvertently altered their minds and ruined them. So human beings went extreme left brained as a result of learning this invention written language and started acting strange. They lost their ability to function with an ecological system and so they became a threat to the ecological system, and they kill off the ecological system and thus kill off their self.

This has nothing to do with saving the environment because mans very nature now is to kill the environment. Mankind is of unsound mind so they cannot save the environment they can only kill it. Mankind does not even know what save the environment even means. Mankind is not capable of understanding the complexity of this situation because the complex aspect of their mind is veiled from the education. There is no solution at all there is only the eventuality. Human beings will kill the ecological system and then they will die and then the ecological system will recover. That is the only eventuality.

So in roughly 5000 years mankind has nearly killed itself off because of this invention which inadvertently altered its mind to extreme left brain. One can take any creature on the planet and alter its mind and that creature will not be viable. That's the law of nature. The mutations get snuffed and that means the mutations their self, snuff their self.

Humans being all across the board all across the world eat too much, have drug addictions, have emotional problems are violent towards each other, are very war prone, are very violent towards other countries or races as it were, this is all a symptom of one thing. Human beings are mentally unsound and they keep pumping out more unsound beings year after year after year and now 5000 years after written language it's starting to show and there is no way to reverse it because the situation is too far gone.

All the wise beings in these ancient were simply saying to the species "You are going to kill yourself off if you do not wake up swiftly." That is all they were saying and now I accidentally wake up and all I can say is enjoy the little time you have left. Do whatever you want to do because it does not matter at all, it is too late. We killed ourselves with this invention because we as a species are mentally unsound as a result of learning this invention and thus we are unviable as a species so we killed our self. I do not want to hear anyone say it matters. Kun huomaan, järkevä ovat aivotoiminnan minä Jumalan Dam muistuttaa. - 9:17:09 AM

9:28:34 AM – How much does your money matter now? How much does you place of worship matter now? How much does your education matter now? How much does your house matter now? How much does your technology matter now? How much does your health matter now? How much do your children matter now? How much does your life matter now? How much does your mind matter now? How much does your wisdom matter now? How much does your government matter now? How much do your friends matter now? How much does your teacher matter now? How much does oxygen matter now? How much does your medicine matter now? How much do your laws matter now? How much does everything you own matter now? How much do your rules matter now? How much do your morals matter now? What is of value now? Who do you say I am now?- 9:31:36 AM

10:37:53 AM – The truth may sound sinister to those who cannot understand it. -10:38:14 AM

10:52:40 AM – The most difficult task of all is trying to convince the sane about population. The sane are in extreme left brain so they are very selfish. They perceive if they do not have offspring they are a failure. The species simply has too many. There are way too many human beings. The sane are in extreme left brain so they only see parts so they see their country as separate from the species so they populate on the premise their country needs more people to compete with countries that have more people than them.

The sane assume all human life is precious and then they assume they should have many children and then they assume it cannot be a bad thing. The sane are unable to grasp anything but sequential logic. One thing leads to another so they take one step at a time and are simply blind to what the next step or ten steps down the road will lead to.

The sane walk towards the cliff but since they are not actually falling yet they assume they are not walking towards the cliff. So the sane see everything as parts and so they only see their self. This is all a left brain sequential symptom. The sequential thoughts given by left brain are good as long as they are kept in mental harmony with the right brains random access thoughts.

Both of these thought aspects are required but the education veils the right random access thoughts so one is left with just sequential thoughts and are thus mentally slothful or at a disadvantage. So when the random access thoughts are veiled one cannot see the end conclusion.   This is what the comment in the religious texts "beginning and the end" and "first and last" denotes in part. First and last is random access. One starts at record 1 and goes to record

100 that is random access in contrast to sequential thoughts that goes from 1 to 2 to 3.

This is what makes the sane mentally unsound, they simply cannot think very far ahead so they tend to repeat the mistakes over and over because they only see one step in front of them. The sane cannot see the whole or all the steps which is what random access is, they only see the next step. This is what mental blindness is. It is not the sane do not have random access because they sane do have a right brain it is simply the education has veiled it and in order to unveil it , it requires a mental technique that goes against what the sane perceive is truth.

This is what the rock and the hard place is. The sane have to defeat the fear that is a symptom of being conditioned into extreme left brain by the education and they cannot do that because they are afraid to do that.

The sane are afraid but they have to not be afraid but they won't be able to do that because they are afraid. The fear is what has to be eliminated but they are too afraid to apply the fear not remedy. So this extreme left brain state is why the population keeps growing and growing. The sane have this god complex where they believe god picked them and so everything revolves around them and so since god picked them they should have as many kids as they can.

The society of the sane actually judge a person on how many kids they have. The families of the sane actually judge their children on whether they have kids or not. So in this left brain state the sane cannot understand the population of perhaps 4 billion too many and then they will say god will work it all out because they do not have the mental capability to grasp the population is a symptom the species is of unsound mind.

This is all relative to me not trying to solve this problem. My mind has already run the numbers and understands there is no solution. The web is too thick at this time to do anything about the problem. Everything is a symptom the species is of unsound mind because of this left brain education and the species continues to educate the next generation with no mental ability to understand why the fear conditioning is required so they do not keep creating more mentally unsound beings. This is why many I speak to who are awake to a degree give up because they perhaps talk their self into some supernatural aspect.

They talk their self into suggesting everyone wakes up eventually so no need to worry. That is a symptom they are not fully awake. They are believing illusions. They do not understand what the tree of knowledge is. They do not fully understand why one has to wake up in the first place. I woke up which denotes I was put to sleep. The absolute reality is none of us should be asleep to begin with but we are put to sleep mentally when we are educated by beings who are asleep and do not realized the importance of the fear conditioning after one gets the written language education. This means unless that weak link is addressed nothing will ever improve ever.

One cannot take a being conditioned into an unsound state of mind and then assume they are going to make anything but unsound decisions. This is just obvious mental psychology. Jos yksi pyytää retard tekemään päätöksen, ja se on jälkeenjäänyt päätöksensä ja kerrottava, että kuusi miljardia olet, mitä meillä nyt tällä planeetalla. Every problem stems back to that one thing, mentally blind people leading mentally blind people. Many will suggest fate and this is how it should be but the truth is, this existence is all a mistake caused by our own invention. We did it to our self and until people understand we really screwed up this time, everything is pointless. The sane are pissing on the tip of the iceberg and cannot figure out what the body of the iceberg even is. So the sane have all their little causes and walk around assuming they are so righteous and at the same time they encourage the children to get the written education and never once suggest the fear not remedy so I have no choice but to spit on all of them because they cannot even wash my feet, psychologically speaking, so to speak. I am begging for you to diagnose me now. This diary is just turning out fantastic.- 11:27:19 AM

Do not assume I have even started to get medieval yet. It is interesting how powerful words are when used against the sane who pray to the demotic. The whole point of all of these diaries is simple. A person who is conditioned into extreme left brain cannot understand these diaries. That is all the proof one needs to understand their random access right brain is veiled. To one in extreme left brain these diaries appear to be babble and to one of sound mind

57

these diaries make perfect sense. If one read this entire diary and comes to the conclusion they cannot understand it that is in reality them proving to their self their right brain random access aspect is essentially non-functioning. I will give the sane infinite proof and they still will doubt. - 11:58:11 AM

1:55:26 PM –   There is no test or experiment one can do to determine if one is mentally exactly in the middle in relation to each hemisphere being active. There are ways to test to see if one is left or right brain is dominate and these are typically traits or deeds one exhibits. In theory one who is in mental harmony should exhibit both characteristics of left and right brain equally. This suggests one who is in the middle or in mental harmony should appear strange to ones with the left brain dominate and with right brain dominate.

Society as a whole has certain rules of etiquette. These rules or expected behavior are in reality forms of conditioning to either right brain to left brain. For example when a parent tells their child to clean their room they are in fact conditioning that child to left brain because left brain is all about organization. Left brain likes to have everything in its proper place and contrary to that right brain is indifferent to organization. This suggests a person that is left brain dominate will see a person in right brain dominate as perhaps lazy or unorganized. A person in left brain will suggest a person in right brain is lazy or unorganized and that is a true observation but it is a characteristic not a flaw. It is not a bad thing it is a trait of one who is right brain dominate to a degree.

One that is right brain dominate will look at all the rules one on the left has and they will perceive that person is very anal retentive with all their rules but that is not bad that is a characteristic of left brain. Left brain loves rules because rules help maintain organization and organization is what left is all about. What this means is a person who is left brain dominate and in a position of authority will slowly start suggesting rules and behaviors and anyone who listens to them will slowly become more left brained. So a parent who is very left brain dominate may throw all these rules at their child and then suggest the child cannot follow rules because the child is lazy or a failure. So the adult in fact mentally conditions that child further into left brain simply because that child is around that adult. Then there is an adult who will comment "My child cannot follow any rules I give it." And they will assume that is because their child is dumb but in reality it is because that adult is so far into left brain and that child is not. So everything that one encounters in all of society in relation to rules or behaviors is in fact encouraging either left or right brain.

The left brain organization aspect appears to be wise but it is really a type of phobia. There are people on the left who cannot stand to have a dirty house. They cannot stand to see one thing out of place so they are far into left brain. They will insult other people who are not as organized as they are. They have this perception in their mind because they are so left brained that if one does not have a perfectly spotless house they are not intelligent. The reality is intelligence is relative to how close one is to being in perfect mental harmony in relation to the two hemisphere of the mind being dominate.

Perfect intelligence would be a person who is 50/50 in relation to both hemispheres being active. Simply put, too far to the right one loses intelligence and too far to the left one loses intelligence. So a sound mind is one that is in the middle. The problem with that is there is no way to measure it because it is on a thought level not a physiological level. The only possible proof is to observe ones deeds or actions or fruits.

The problem with that is if a person is in extreme left brain or extreme right brain the deeds and actions of one in perfect mental harmony will appear abnormal. The ones in extreme left brain perceive what they think is normal is absolute normal and the same with ones in extreme right brain. For example one in mental harmony has moment of organization but it is not their life goal to be organization or they can survive if there is not always organization.

One in extreme left brain cannot stand disorganization for more than a moment. When one is too far to the left this organization aspect is a flaw. One in extreme left brain cannot stand disorganization so that is their weakness and change or uncertain events are disorganization and so they do not do well in those situations. Change bothers one in extreme left brain because it is uncertain and its is unknown and so the unknown is their weakness.

Contrary to left brain one in right brain flourishes with unknowns and change. The disorganization is really adaptation. One in left brain who has everything organized, and then something unexpected happens and they panic.

If a mind has no difficulties with disorganization or what could be called chaos then they can adapt to any situation and if one is very organization centered they cannot adapt to chaos well. So a person who is very left brained loses their job and that denotes chaos or unknown and they panic and go home and kill their self. That is a good example of one who cannot adapt to chaos or uncertain situations. That person got a bomb shell dropped on them and they panicked and did something stupid. That is the flaw of organization or being in the extreme left brain state.

The basis of society is based on organization, rules and structure and that is all left brained. So when the slightest unknown factor is thrown into that machine the machine breaks down because the minds that control that machine are so far left brained they cannot adapt to chaos well. A person who gets lost in the wilderness is faced with chaos and the ones who do best are the ones who have some degree of right brain still active. The ones that panic and make mistakes are the ones who are so far left brained that situation of disorganization and unknown defeats them. Society as a whole is left brained and so society as a whole hates change and does not do well with adaptation.

It is not a matter of what the change is, it is a matter that change suggests disorganization and left brain loves organization. So society is left brained and conditioned into left brain and then makes rules and more rules and goes further into left brain with the belief that rules create organization. Rules do not create organization it is simply the left brain majority perceive rules create organization. Rules create isolation. Isolation suggests parts and labels and that is also a trait of left brain.

The aspect of rules denotes if you break a rule you are deemed bad and if you follow the rules you are conditioned further into left brain. This is simply a symptom every single thing someone says to you that you should or should not do is really conditioning a person into right or left brain. A child hangs around friends and they say

"Screw the adults and their rules" and so that child is conditioned to right brain a little and then that child goes home to the adults and the adults say "Clean your room or you get punished." and that conditions the child back to the left and so mentally the child is being ripped apart by these two forces. Soon the child gets confused and one side wins out. Eventually the adults may tell that child to never hang around those kids for they are a bad influence so the adults win in their left brain conditioning of that child. The adults have the leverage, the punishments and have the fear tactics to make sure that child falls in line with the adults perceived ideal that if a person has enough rules and organization they will be wise when in reality all they will be is extreme left brained.- 2:44:53 PM

5:16:02 PM – A person from civilization who has the education and thus is very left brained. They go to one of these tribes that does not have the education so these tribes have a pretty strong right brain still. The left brain person first notices the tribes do not make the children wear shoes. So already the left brain person starts to panic. They already feel sorry for the children because they don't have shoes on and so they want to rescue the children. The left brain person has these rules in their head and if the rules are broken it is evil or bad to them. What mentally is happening is a left brain person is a salve to all of these rules and when the rules are broken they feel unsafe and they stress out and get angry. They are essentially walking time bombs looking for rules being broken. It is not even important to them what the rules are, all they understand is the rules create organization and without organization they have chaos and they cannot handle chaos or uncertainty because that is the strength of the right brain and their right brain is veiled.

One can look at the habits of a pack of monkeys and understand there are no rules. That is why they are considered to be in the wild. Wild denotes no organization. There are no rules in nature relative to behavior there are only many left brained people who perceive rules are needed to keep organization. If the tribes who live in the wild had any flaws they wouldn't be alive. They are alive and have been living like that for thousands of years so this left brain person goes there and see's all these perceives rules in their head being broken and they want to fix the tribes.

The ones on the left are simply nervous wrecks because they are so left brained they cannot tolerate uncertainty. The ones on the left hate anyone who hates rules so they hate anyone on the right simply because their minds in extreme left brain keeps telling them without rules you have no organization and then you are in danger and danger is relative to fear. So the more danger they perceive the more rules they need and the more nervous they become when the rules are broken. The rules are totally irrelevant, the fact their rules are being broken is what the problem is. So then there is this situation where the ones on the left with all of their rules determine anyone on the right who doesn't like rules is bad or evil because they are not like them. The ones on the left only have one thing in their mind "What rules do you subscribe to."

The ones on the left try to call them morals or standards or accepted norms but they are not morals or accepted norms they are benchmarks so they can tell who is evil and who is good. That is also relative to left brain categorizing everything or seeing parts. It does not matter if it's political or religious beliefs these beliefs are simply rules and if one does not adhere to them they certainly must be evil. So there is a whole world of left brainers and each group or country has their rules and any country that does not agree with their rules is deemed evil.

The left brainers logic is simply if you do not follow the rules I follow you are evil so a right brain person comes along and says I do not follow all of those rules and they are deemed evil and punished. This all leads up to true racism.

Society educates people and they inadvertently go left brain so the whole world is left brain and prone to wanting tons of rules so they feel safe and not afraid and they hold everyone who is not left brain captive or under their power or control structure. The left brainers will suggest you need infinite rules to be safe and so everything is organized and that is not true in absolute terms only in their left brain state of mind.

Other words their suggestion that rules create organization and thus safety is a lie. It is all in their head, It is all relative to their extreme left brain mental state, it is not truth in absolute terms. So the lefters are running around pushing all their rules on people and assuming they are righteous to do so but in reality they are just control freaks with an unsound minds or way too far into left brain. The left brain people are not satisfied with ten rules they want as many rules as they can because they perceive rules create safety and they are fear based so they perceives rules will keep them safe. The rules they want have no end because the perceive the more rules they have the better. That is what left brain is all about, rules. The lefter's will try to suggest we need some rules but they are unable to grasp they only want infinite rules so they will feel organized and safe. The control freaks and their rule delusions always win because they can always tell someone on the left "That person broke the rules so they are evil." and that person on the left will agree because they love rules too.

The left brainer's minds are so dark because they only look for rules being broken. They say "He did drugs he is evil.", "He cussed he is evil.", "He misspelled a word he is evil." That is all their whole life is, looking for rules being broken so they can scold the rule breakers so they feel safe and organized. The only solution is to divide the world up into right brain people and left brain people and that way the left brain people can make rules until they are all in little cages and the right brain people can enjoy no rules because if that is not the case then one mental group dominates the other mental group and that is slavery. - 5:44:59 PM

6:00:55 PM – The cerebral point of all of this is when a society conditions people with written education into extreme left brain, then makes all of these rules knowing the left brain beings they have conditioned love the rules, then throws anyone who breaks their infinite rules in jail and in cages or discriminates against ones who do not get enough of their education, then dooms these beings to slave jobs and disadvantages, society is really racist against right brain.

6:26:12 PM – The last I checked I just sit in my isolation chamber writing these stupid diaries so I understand I have this strange mental sensation that I have been mentally raped and my life was taken from me mentally speaking from this left brain conditioning but I cannot grasp how long forty years is any longer so I have no ability to gauge how much it cost me. I can't say it cost me money because money or material things do not give me satisfaction or dissatisfaction. I cannot say I was robbed of a physical thing and I am unable to really tell what I was robbed of. I cannot suggest I was robbed of my life because in the last ten months with no sense of time it seems like eternity so that is not a good argument. So I am always reduced back to a neutral mindset. First I have to talk myself out of writing these infinite diaries, but perhaps if I do that I will have to write infinite books explaining why I am no longer writing infinite diaries.

I cannot figure out how Moses killed people, that one person he buried in the sand and then the army, the red sea story. It must have been so difficult for him to do that because the cerebral heightened awareness is so powerful it is just like the Incas when they saw the Spanish. The Incas said the Spanish were gods. The reason this state of mind is bad is because this whole world is full of left brain wolves who will rape you into hell if you trust them, and when you feel them with the vision aspect you will trust them. You can't trust the dust. They have no eyes. - 6:40:54 PM

Happiness is fleeting so it is really a stage of sorrow but neutral can be maintained.

9/9/2009 11:11:24 AM – I want to make one thing very clear. I am now in another world mentally and the only way to describe how I recall I was for nearly forty years would be, in mental hell. It is not even important what exactly this state of mind I am in now even is. Somehow when I accidentally got all the fear out of my mind and I could do the one thing I could never do with that strong sense of time, strong emotions, strong cravings, strong desires and strong sense of hunger for all those years and that is think clearly.

There is not enough material wealth in the universe that can compare to being able to think clearly. I do not need anyone to tell me what to think because I can think for myself and that comment alone is perhaps beyond the ability of the sane to even grasp. Thinking for one's self is perhaps a scary proposition to some but it is what freedom really is all about. Life is an equation that requires one to have all their mental faculties working at full power at all times and fear in the mind is what negates that possibility.

What really starts the mental cycle of one starting to think for their self is when one decides to apply this fear not conditioning because it goes against the logic of everyone on the left. There is perhaps no one on the left who will suggest this fear not conditioning is safe, logical or sane but the moment a person on the left ignores that universal opinion they start to think for their self and they stop subscribing to the opinions of the herd for perhaps the first time in their life.

One gets to a point mentally where they ask their self a question. One hears the experts on the left suggest this fear not conditioning is crazy then one thinks "Maybe all these experts on the left are crazy."

To one on the left this fear not conditioning appears very harsh and if one perceives it is not harsh they perhaps are not grasping what it is suggesting but to ones who have applied it is like falling off a log. It is simply a mental decision one makes under stress. One on the left perceives death is near and they go against the grain of that left brain fear and this silences that left brain back to it normal level.

It is strictly a mental intangible decision that takes one second yet it changes everything mentally for that person forever. That one second mental decision does not perhaps burn any calories so it cannot even be measured in the realm of physical effort and so this decision is beyond the scale of measure. This one second decision in fact defies E=Mc2 because one in reality gets so much for nothing. That one second decision under perceived stress is intangible on every level so it is nothing. One gets into a situation of perceived death and makes a mental decision not to run and thus submit to that perceived death and their perception of everything changes, yet nothing has really happened on the scale of physical change. The point is, it does not cost anything. This event does not take a lifetime it takes one split second. One can spend their whole life looking for a materialistic nirvana or they can make a split second decision based on a thought level and surpass the value of all material wealth. Who told you that you aren't the wise man? I never told you that you aren't the wise man. - 11:59:11 AM

1:28:23 PM – There is in fact no law on the books against mental abuse. This left brain education conditioning if not administered properly with the proper fear or attachment conditioning to counteract the left brain written language condition leaves one's mind drastically altered. There is no law against doing that to an adult or a child and that adult or child may not even be aware that has happened to them because when the education is administered they were a child and their mind was not fully developed to begin with.

I find it difficult to imagine any human being would intentionally do that to another human being and I try to stay out of the supernatural realm so I am at this crossroad where I try to figure out if human beings are that sinister or if human beings are blind to the fact they are that sinister. I am far past the point of doubting that the sequential based written education in fact is conditioning people to extreme left brain. That is an understood variable at this point. That is now a fact beyond all facts. If it is a manmade intentional invention to keep people mentally unsound and thus makes people easy to control and thus easily prone to fear tactics then the only solution is an all out war in every definition of the word war. Simply put a no morals, no sympathy, no mercy kind of war. Total carnage would be an accurate description.

On the other hand if this is just a misunderstanding in relation to an invention that has unintended consequences mentally speaking on anyone who gets this education then it can be explained and humans will adapt to that explanation and attempt to remedy the unintended consequences. It is one thing to be ignorant about a situation and then that ignorance causes suffering but one is not aware it is causes suffering and it is another thing for one to intentionally make others suffer and knowingly so.

Then there is the supernatural aspect and I mean supernatural as in a force on a mental scale or a mental influence that manipulates people to control them and this written education would be that catalyst for the supernatural aspect to control a person thoughts and once a person thoughts are controlled their deeds or fruits can be controlled or manipulated. I do not detect a whole lot of peace, love, and happiness would be the bullet point of this section of my poorly disguised diary. I do not detect if I spell my words properly and use commas properly it is going to help me in this situation. It is perhaps a bit more complex than just putting the letters in proper sequence. Perhaps the sane assume spelling a word in proper sequence is what complexity is.

Perhaps the only thing the sane have relative to complexity is their inability to detect complexity. I would rather be writing about some UFO that is coming to attack earth or some ghost that is going to attack us than to write about the fact this sequential heavy and rule heavy written language invention is indirectly conditioning anyone who gets that education into extreme left brain and thus altering their minds for their entire life. I would rather not suggest we are out own worst enemy but we are our own worst enemy. Aliens coming from mars is much more believable than this demotic induce neurosis. I would rather write about the prospects of walking on the water and turning a stick into a snake than writing about the reality of demotic induced neurosis. The sane have trouble believing this condition happened to them as a child because it would destroy their entire safety system in their mind. It would turn everything they think about everything upside down. I will tell the sane I am an accident and I accidentally broke this curse and I did not mean to it was just an accident I could not foresee and if they believed that then their next conclusion would be, if it happened to you because of the education then it happen to me.

This is all relative to one who gets abused tends to protect or sympathize with the one who abused them. That is relative to self esteem. Self esteem is relative to being in extreme left brain from the education. Self esteem is really pride. Pride is ego and one in extreme left brain has huge ego characteristics. Simply put they have trouble swallowing crow.

I am in fact not talking about myself I am in fact telling six billion people they have been mentally put to sleep as a result of being educated with written language. If it was intentional or unintentional it still does not change the bottom line that one is mentally asleep.

When society detects a person who is destroying and damaging others and the environment directly or indirectly with no regards to those around them, they lock them up, so to speak.

I am suggesting there are six billion human beings going around destroying and damaging others and their self and the environment around them with no regards to those around them. The very ones who doubt that are the ones I am talking about. The very ones who deny that are the ones I am talking about. The very ones who control the herd are the ones I am talking about. I am either the most crazy human being in the universe and in all of history or I am telling the truth and that truth is far beyond the sane beings understanding. I am not going to preach peace. I am not going to preach kindness. I am not going to preach mercy. I am not going to preach compassion. I will leave those topics to the ones who are looking to make a buck. - 2:12:03 PM

[Acts 28:3 And when Paul had gathered a bundle of sticks, and laid them on the fire, there came a viper out of the heat, and fastened on his hand.] - I could not have said it better myself. I have more viper bites on my right hand than I am able to explain with words.

Ich kenne thy Arbeiten und Drangsal und Armut, (aber Tausendkunstreiche) und ich wissen, dass die Blasphemie von ihnen, welche sie sagen fromm sind und nicht sind, aber die Synagoge von Satan sind. I am quite certain I have blown it now. - 3:03:48 PM

What I detect psychologically here is the ones on the left only see things as parts. That the problem. Here is an example.
[2 Timothy 1:7 For God hath not given us the spirit of fear; but of power, and of love, and of a sound mind.]

Mind is the same thing as spirit. If one has an unsound mind they have an unsound spirit and if one has an unsound spirit they have an unsound mind. The symptom of an unsound mind is fear, any fear. Ones on the left only see's parts so mind and spirit are not the same thing at all to them.

Here is another example:

[Ephesians 5:5 For this ye know, that no whoremonger, nor unclean person, nor covetous man, who is an idolater, hath any inheritance in the kingdom of Christ and of God.]

An unclean person is a person with an unsound mind. This is not suggesting a person who has dirty hands or has dirt on them it is suggesting psychology. Unsound mind is a mind with fear in it and fear is a symptom one has been conditioned far to the left mentally by the written education which is sequential based and that is left brain. The next part of this comment is covetous man or idolater. That is not a judgment that is a symptom psychologically of a person in extreme left brain. Covet denotes one who craves material things because their cerebral powerhouse right brain is veiled. Idolater is the same thing. Mohammed said "The Jews and Christians make shrines out of the graves of their prophets." What that means is, the ones who heard the remedy from Moses and Abraham and Jesus which is fear not, never applied it so they are showing symptoms mentally they did not apply it. They are still physically or materialistically focused and that means their right brain cerebral powerhouse is veiled.

Once the powerhouse right brain is unveiled one becomes very cerebral and so that means the left brain materialistic aspect becomes veiled. So one who suggests they are a Jew or Christian or Muslim but has not applied the hard core submit to fear, fear not, those who lose their life will preserve it remedy to the tree of knowledge are everything in the universe but a Jew a Christian or a Muslim. The last I checked I am not a Jew a Christian or a Muslim, I am an accident. An accident is an event one was not expecting.

[2 Peter 3:10 But the day of the Lord will come as a thief in the night; in the which the heavens shall pass away with a great noise, and the elements shall melt with fervent heat, the earth also and the works that are therein shall be burned up.]

Perhaps there is no need to clarify this comment.

So the ancient texts are codes they are only decipherable by ones who have applied the fear not remedy and they are undecipherable to ones who have not. Simply put the key to these codes is relative to your mind. If one's mind is in extreme left brain they only see parts and so they get a totally different interpretation of these codes totally in every way. Once the right brain is unveiled then one gets the spirit or sees the whole of the code the code is easily understood. This comment explains that.

[Daniel 9:13 As it is written in the law of Moses, all this evil is come upon us: yet made we not our prayer before the LORD our God, that we might turn from our iniquities, and understand thy truth.]

"All this evil is come upon us". This is complex but from a psychological point of view one can understand the written language conditions people into left brain extreme and makes their deeds or fruits sour. From a supernatural point of view a sinister aspect suggested man invent this written language as a way to infest mans spirit or mind with evil and so a man's fruits or deeds are sour. Whichever is the case the same situation exists because the mind is unsound at the end of the day because of the fear instilled by the education.

Ones on the left tend to try to take things to a logical conclusion but they are unable to do that because their thoughts are sequential. They go two steps and assume that is the logical conclusion. That is the nature of sequential thought and sequential thought is left brained. They think if they cannot take it any further than they have that must be the logical conclusion but the reality is sequential thoughts do not go very far and also do not go very fast and that is what sloth is all about. Sequential thoughts are sloth in contrast to the powerhouse unnamable right brain which processes at random access speed. One can never argue with that reality. Ones who understand what random access is will never argue that sequential access is faster. The contrast is like night and day and dark and light, and so this all lead's to this comment:

[that we might turn from our iniquities, and understand thy truth.]

Turn from our iniquities is the same thing as repent and repent is a onetime thing which is simply the remedy to the left brain conditioning and that is fear not or fear conditioning and then one will understand the truth. So this is saying unless one applies the remedy to the left brain conditioning education enabled one will never understand the truth because their mind in that extreme left brain state is the bottle neck. One will always see parts and have sequential thoughts and so they can never see the truth and understand the code in these texts because the code in these texts requires random access thought and seeing things as a whole and that's right brain. I am not talking about psychology, philosophy, or spirituality. I am talking about the light, the truth, the way. - 3:49:12 PM

[Acts 26:27 King Agrippa, believest thou the prophets? I know that thou believest.]

This is a revealing comment because it is Paul saying to the King, don't you believe what Abraham and Moses said about the covenant which is fear not? Paul is saying he is not suggesting a new concept he is suggesting what the ones 500 years before him suggested. This is the key to everything because Paul and Jesus were not bringing a new message they were repeating what Moses and Abraham said is the remedy to this left brain conditioning which is fear not or fear conditioning. Then Mohammed came 500 years after this and said I agree with Moses and with Jesus and then altered fear not to be submit (to fear) and they were all on the same page. But the ones on the left only see things as parts so it turned into a huge religious war and a nightmare. So never assume anyone got the message because the last I checked the sane are all still killing each other and spitting in the face of these wise beings in the process- 4:49:13 PM

4:52:03 PM – To clarify everything I have ever written. When one is in a situation where they perceive death or harm in a mental sense not in an actual sense, a mental sense would be one perceives a ghost in the night is going to get them, an actual sense is when one in the water is surrounded by sharks, and they do not run from it , they submit to it , thus submit.

So we have a person who perceives death or harm in a mental sense and that left brain is fear, I will explain why the fear is great soon, so it is saying "Run like the wind danger is coming". What one does when they do not run is they fear not or they lose their life and preserve it or they submit to that perceived danger. So this is all a mental head game.

The left brain is way to strong and it is making one afraid of things that are not an actual threat to them. That is what a hallucination is. One is in fact mentally hallucinating if they are in the dark and thinking something supernatural is going to harm them, one is simply believing hallucinations.

Psychologically speaking, when one reacts to hallucinations they are mentally unsound and also a danger to their self and those around them. You go tell your shrink when you sat in a cemetery at night you sensed a ghost was going to kill you and so you ran away and they will perhaps put you on some very heavy drugs because you are mentally unstable if they don't it is probably because they would have run also.

So perhaps you shouldn't be going to a shrink who believes in hallucinations like you do. One who is prone to hallucinations is perhaps not the best choice to assist one who is prone to hallucinations. Some on the left will suggest "You need fear to survive". I am suggesting that comment is a lie. Common sense and fear are not the same thing. One who runs from what they perceive is a ghost in a cemetery at night is afraid, and automatically they lose common sense.

72

[2 Timothy 1:7 For God hath not given us the spirit of fear; but of power, and of love, and of a sound mind.] This comment was made 2000 years ago and it suggests fear is not real or fear is not required to live, and also suggests not everyone fears, namely ones of sound mind. So whoever suggested fear is needed and fear is real is in fact suggesting this comment made 2000 years ago is a lie.

I accidentally found out this spirit of fear is a symptom of an unsound mind because I have no fear and that means I can think clearly without the fear getting in the way so I do not have this emotion fear.

There is a story about some men who went to an island and found some new species of animals, one was a giant rat. The men commented the rats were not afraid of man and so the rats did not run from man. So this shows fear is often confused with common sense. Fear is not needed to understand one should not walk out in front of a Mac truck that in fact is the realm of common sense. The more fear one has the more fear based decisions one makes and the less common sense decisions one makes.

What I suggest is I accidentally understand now what fear not means in this comment made 2500 years ago.

[Genesis 15:1 After these things the word of the LORD came unto Abram in a vision, saying, Fear not, Abram: I am thy shield, and thy exceeding great reward.]

I am not preaching supernatural because if you have the fear in your head the last thing in the universe you want me to start talking about is supernatural. If you have that fear in your head because you have not applied fear not after getting the education you are mentally unable to handle what I understand about supernatural so I avoid that topic for your sake. I pride myself in failing one sentence at a time.- 5:15:41 PM

5:27:11 PM – The most complex thing about all of this is not about me trying to reach people who already have the conditioning. I can suggest strong sense of time, strong hunger, strong emotions and fear are in fact a symptom of the extreme left brain conditioning into infinity, but people will ask their friends who are also conditioned if that is true and they will say "No everyone has strong emotions, strong sense of time, strong hunger and fear so that is normal."

The reality is a crazy person will see another crazy person as sane and in turn see a sane person as crazy. Here is all I hear in religious chat rooms day in and day out.

<TwYsTeD`> your babel needs to stop

I get this impression mentally that I really cannot reach the adults because they are too far gone or they have been in left brain extreme since they were very young and they no longer can tell what being mentally sound is.

The reality is I am a failed suicide and that denotes I came close enough to think I was dying from all the pills and I made peace with death and did not call for help. This means it is impossible I meant for this to happen, this waking up. Some suggest there are no accidents but it was an accident. It does not satisfy me to explain these ideas and it does not dissatisfy me because mentally I am in neutral. I am not on a crusade. I simply understand children are being mentally raped and I am trying to address that understanding with words. - 5:40:11 PM

[2 Timothy 1:7 For God hath not given us the spirit of fear; but of power, and of love, and of a sound mind.]

I cannot prove to you that fear is a symptom of an unsound mind and thus a symptom of an unsound spirit. If one has fear in their mind and thus in their spirit it was not put there by God or nature. One can define god any way they want but it will never change the fact that God did not put that fear in you. So then the next conclusion is "What did put that fear in me?" The answer to that is something not of God or nature. This something not of God, whatever you think it is, has a calling card, and it is called fear. So fear is symptom that something not of God is in one's mind or spirit. I prefer to suggest the written language education has made people very left brain dominate and a side effect of that is this fear aspect but I will also add I believe what Timothy said is absolute truth. I detect the spirit of truth about what Timothy said about this fear.

Later on in this passage Timothy suggests the word gentiles. Ones on the left are usually thinking about physical aspects as opposed to

74

cerebral aspects. This is why it is important to understand a gentile is not relative to genetics or physical aspects at all. A gentile is one who got the education and did not apply the fear not remedy, relative to this time period and location in the world a Jew is one who did apply the fear not remedy.

[2 Timothy 1:11 Whereunto I am appointed a preacher, and an apostle, and a teacher of the Gentiles.]

This is Timothy saying he is a Jew because he applied the fear not remedy and he is trying to assist the ones who have not yet applied it, or teaching them how to apply it, and they are known as gentiles. This is a good example how the ones on the left only see parts. They miss the inside information in the texts. Timothy is not saying right out he is Jew but he is saying he is a teacher of the Gentiles which denotes he is a Jew. A gentile does not teach a gentile because they are both Gentiles. A Jew does not teach a Jew because they are both Jews.

It is very difficult to reach the ones on the left because they see the parts and they never assume one part is the same as another part. A person who applies fear not relative to this time period and location is Jew and also a Christian and 500 years later they were called Muslims and in the east around Moses time they were called Buddha and relative to Socrates time period and location they were called philosophers. Ones on the left perhaps cannot grasp that because that means their definitions of all these words are wrong and their strong pride and ego which is a symptom of being left brain to an extreme will make them say things like "That is crazy and wrong and a lie."

What is amazing is this written education altered our minds to such a degree we can actually assume another human being is not a human being, that a symptom of the labels left brain encourages. A human being is a human being and the minute a human being gets this extreme left brain conditioning they may suggest another human being is not a human being and so they are in fact hallucinating. The only difference in how human beings act is the mind.

A human being conditioned into left brain by education will never have the fruits of a human being who has countered that extreme left brain state of mind. So there is a mental difference and there are explainable symptoms to the mental differences. Some describe these psychological characteristics as sin of the flesh and some describe them as psychological states of mind but the point is they are indicative to ones state of mind in relation to being extreme left brained or being in mental harmony or of sound mind.

There are too many symptoms to deny and some call them the fruits of the tree which means the characteristics of the mind, or how one acts. The Native Americans lived in harmony for thousands of years and then the ones who got the education arrived and essentially destroyed everything in their path in short order and thus one can contrast the fruits of these two cultures of human beings. One culture lived in harmony and one culture killed all the beavers for 50 bucks. This is all an indication of the contrary mental state these two cultures were in. The underlying difference is one culture did not have written language and one culture did. - 6:31:28 PM

9/10/2009 2:16:28 AM – Age is not relative to wisdom or common sense.

I submit I am sloppy because I cannot seem to sleep so I am going to translate some random stuff.

[Proverbs 28:5 Evil men understand not judgment: but they that seek the LORD understand all things.]

"Evil men understand not judgment" this comment is first off what speaking in tongues is. It appears strange to ones on the left. Evil men are the ones on the left who got the education and did not apply the fear not remedy. "Understand not judgment" denotes they do not agree with or understand what fear not really means. "But they that seek the Lord" Lord is the remedy. The remedy is to face ones fear as in fear not and the full measure of that is to face ones fear of death or perceived death, then the right hemisphere unveils and one understands all things.

The "understand all things" denotes the extreme power the right brain has when it is unveiled. Right brain is unnamable in power. I do not understand how I understand all the things I do understand since the accident so I just have to say right brain power is unnamable. Right brain when unveiled is beyond measure because even the person with it unveiled cannot fully grasp its power. It is simply spooky.

9/10/2009 2:22:37 PM – I woke up today and thought I should never tell people these things because they might achieve this state of mind and maybe it's bad so I have quite a lot of ambiguity or doubt at times. To me it's funny because I am aware right brain has lots of ambiguity so when I have it I just ignore it because I understand that's expected. That's kind of why all these wise ones failed at times because they were so full of doubt. My logic in relation to the fear not methods is "Make sure you reach this state of mind but maybe you shouldn't." So once a person is conditioned into left brain they have these people who have tons of doubt by nature of the right brain being unveiled trying to convince them to go back to sound mind. It is not doubt about basic things it is more about doubt in relation to if this state of mind is proper and that is because one is mentally in neutral. Suggesting this state of mind is neutral freaks people out who are use to the highs and lows. - 2:30:13 PM

4:09:27 PM – It's hard to persuade my old friend we are friends. - 4:09:43 PM

9:41:54 PM - unus ut est minimus evinco bestia -9:42:03 PM

9/11/2009 1:57:01 AM -Left brain is sequential based right brain is random access based, think about language, abc's that's sequential. 123 that's sequential. Spelling words is arranging letters in proper sequence, addition and subtraction is sequential based. After years of this education the mind is totally left brain and thus the right brain is veiled and like a crescent moon. This is not on a physiological level, this is a mental conditioning. Thoughts are not tangible so this conditioning is not even measureable so the only way to determine how far one is thrown into left brain is to look for symptoms. Behavior patterns. Mental symptoms.

When a person misspells a word in school a teacher judges the student or grades that student. This judgment or grade either rewards the student for getting the sequence right or punishes the student for getting the sequence wrong and in this case spells the word properly or not. A student understands early on if they spell enough words in sequence properly they will be praised by the teacher and their parents. This is elementary mental conditioning, rewards for good conditioning and punishment for bad conditioning. The carrot on the stick is based on the premise if you spell enough words in sequence you get good grades and then when you get older you get a good job and thus lots of money and an easy life. The actual reality is, if you spell enough words properly you condition your mind into such extreme left brain you alter your mind and thoughts to such an extreme you become mentally imbalanced.

So written language and reading and math are nothing more than brainwashing tools, no drugs required. The drug is the lure of easy money at the end of the tunnel and an easy life and acceptance by your friends and parents and peers and society. This means all of society is complicit in mentally conditioning children into this extreme left brain state of mind which in fact mentally ruins children. The parents had it done to them and the leaders had it done to them and the religious leaders had it done to them and everyone had it done to them going all the way back in history. Even in the realm of recorded history 2000 BC, even at that time the known world was conditioned into the extreme left brain state of mind except for the tribes. Recorded history itself is a symptom of the neurosis mankind was conditioned into. Recorded history itself is simply a record of when mankind conditioned itself into neurosis.

The pyramids are a symptom mankind went mentally bad and started building in vain attempts to show pride and ego. The wars are a symptom of beings being in left brain to an extreme and thus only seeing things as parts. This is the us against them mentality. Desires and craving to gain material things such as the control of recourses and gold and are all a symptoms of a human who is into such extreme left brain they started doing things that were nothing more than a symptom of a creature that is very mentally unbalanced.

After this conditioning human beings needed lots of food to eat because their sense of hunger was greatly increased. Human beings needed much more food than they needed before the conditioning and so food became scarce. Humans had to start growing food when before there was plenty of food to eat just by wandering around and picking food off the tree that grew naturally. There was no such thing as eating more than once a day until after the neurosis. The vast increase in hunger also caused many physiological problems. Obesity is an obvious symptom but also the body itself had to evolve to compensate for this large food intake on a daily basis.

The large amount of food that a human in neurosis perceives they need to eat also cause the organs such as the liver and the kidneys and the digestive system to evolve.

The very nervous system was also altered so the humans in neurosis were very nervous and frightened and embarrassed and essentially they were a ball of nerves. This also created great stress on the physiological aspects of the body. This great change in nervousness enabled many new diseases to start showing up in the body. The perceived stress caused by this mentally unsound state of mind was enough to affect the immune system and so this left brain conditioning in fact caused many diseases than humans had never experienced before.

So in short mankind invented written language and math and this lead to the extreme left brain neurosis and then many symptoms of this mental imbalance started showing up but were perceived by the ones in neurosis to be symptoms they were becoming smarter, or more aware of things but in reality they were symptoms something had gone terribly wrong, but they could not figure that out because they were in fact mentally unable to figure that out because the complex right brain that is best at detecting patterns had been veiled to such an extreme they were mentally unaware to think properly or detect these patterns and symptoms.

This neurosis is similar to what happens to a person when they are on very heavy drugs like PCP. The person believes what they perceive is real. The humans perceived this strong hunger was just a normal characteristic because everyone around then in the neurosis also had great hunger. The human's perceived sense of time was normal because all the ones in neurosis around them also had strong sense of time. The human's perceived fear was normal because all the ones in neurosis around them had fear. So the neurosis was transmitted by teaching more people this written language and Math and slowly everyone started to fall under this neurosis. In short order perhaps within a thousand years after the inventions, vast majority of the people were in this mental neurosis. This was enabled because the written language and math were looked at as a sign of intelligence and thus power.

The wise men of the time were thought to be the ones who had the most education when in fact that was only relative to the ones in neurosis. It was thought the more education one had the smarter they were so the more power they had and this encouraged more people to want to get the education. So this education was in fact self perpetuating. Once a parent got the education and thus fell under the neurosis they would teach it to their children and this cycle was never broken. The adults taught it to the children and the children taught it to their children and so all of the symptoms of being in the neurosis became norms. The strong hunger became a norm when in reality it was an abnormality. The strong fear and emotions became a norm when in fact they were an abnormality. The many diseases and physiological symptoms were considered norms when they were in fact abnormalities. The emotional problems were considered normal when in fact they were abnormal. Suicides and depression were considered just a part of life when in fact they were direct symptoms of this extreme left brain neurosis.

All of these problems were symptoms of the neurosis but the ones in neurosis just assumed they were new problems that needed to be addressed and so when they were addressed they only created more problems. The strong hunger created the need to grow crops so then they needed to make irrigation systems to grow enough food to feed everyone and when they could not do it people starved so the starvation was also an indirect symptom of the neurosis.

The left brain neurosis simply changed the human beings entire behavior. The human cravings for material things was so drastic the ones who were not at the top of the control structure had to steal to get enough food and enough wealth to survive, so to arrived crime and with the crime became laws, and with the laws became punishment and jail.

All of these inventions were simply ways to counter act all the problems that the neurosis was causing. Even after the first thousand years after the written language and math inventions it was too late to reverse the neurosis that learning these sequential based inventions caused. The human beings who were still living normally and were not subjugated to the neurosis were unable to remedy the situation simply because they were quite docile in contrast to the ones in neurosis. The human beings not mentally unsound were not able to defeat the ones in neurosis because they were not violent by nature in a sound state of mind so they tried the best they could to avoid the ones in neurosis who lived in what were called cities or civilization.

The ones in neurosis looked upon the ones who lived in the wilderness as lower life forms because the ones in neurosis saw the ones in neurosis around them as normal when in reality the ones still in the wilderness were normal or of sound mind. The lambs could not defeat the lions because the lambs were not violent or adapt at war in contrast to the lions, the ones in neurosis. This was a determining factor in ensuring the neurosis could not be controlled or reversed.

Eventually the ones in neurosis started using up all the resources and so they needed to take more and more land and control more and more water sources to keep feeding the ever growing populations that the cities produced.

The population growth was also a symptom of the neurosis. The humans in neurosis could no longer think clearly so they had children even when they could not maintain a steady food supply for the children they had. The left brain extreme state they were in made them lose the ability to think as a whole and they could only see parts so all the families in the cities only saw their family as important and so they all had this goal to only think about their own family with no regard to the other families.

The neurosis caused each family to grow in size until the entire city was over populated so they had to branch out to a new area and create another city and find new water supplies and new food sources because of their great appetite for food caused by the neurosis. The ones in neurosis being only able to see parts started to think of their self as the most important animal. They started to think of their family as the most important family. They started killing off other families and other kinds of animals because they could only see their own self as important and their own family as important so they lost their sense of harmony.

This neurosis caused the humans to develop a strong ego and thus a strong pride so they all thought of their self as this supreme ruler or supreme life form in not only contrast to all other animals but also in contrast to ones who were not like them or in contrast to ones in the wilderness who were not in neurosis.

The ones in neurosis could only see things in parts so they also saw other cities as enemies or not equals and this also included different races of humans and also different cultures. The ones in neurosis could only see their self as important and everyone else around them as unimportant in contrast. This also led to even the parents looking at their own children as not being equals so the parents even hated their own children or were displeased with their own offspring and this was also a symptom of the mentally unsound state of mind they were in from the education.

All of these symptoms along with the strong emotions caused many to seek ways to escape all of these problems and also escape the nervousness the neurosis was causing. This need to relieve the extreme nervousness lead the humans in neurosis to start taking many different kinds of drugs. Some of these drugs helped them partially escape the mental neurosis for a short while caused by the education. The drugs relived the nervousness but it also created many problems as a result so these problems kept multiplying all because of the written language and math induced neurosis. - 3:14:16 AM

4:27:07 AM - EGO have nondum exorsus scribo , pugno , habeo os.- 4:28:34 AM

9:51:59 AM – Civilization does not like thinkers it likes consumers who do not think. - 9:52:29 AM

7:42:51 PM – A judge seeks retribution an observer seeks understanding.

When the vast majority of the people are in this extreme left brain state and can only see
parts they cannot function as a group because they only see their self. These labels that they are inclined to, run so deep, they always end up on their own mission. First they are humans then they are of a country of origin, then they are of a specific belief system, like a religion or a lack of religion, then they are of a specific political point of view, then they are of are of a particular race, then they are of a particle class in relation to economic stability or financial aspects. Even with all of these labels they still perceive they are the number one priority so to speak. For example even in a club or religious situation there are conflicts.
Even when a person is a part of a club they dislike other people in that club. Even in a relationship they cannot get along with their mate. They cannot get alone with their offspring because they perceive they know best. There is a group of fifty people and they all know the best because they are in such extreme left brain they see everything as parts. This means even when they find something they like they tend to eventually turn against it. They will suggest every human life is sacred but in reality they are really saying is life that is not human is not important or sacred. That is a god complex. This is symptom this left brain state of mind has thrown their thoughts into a realm that they can no longer determine what is reality. It is

not possible humans can be the most important life form because if all other life forms were taken away humans would die and so that means human beings are simply another aspect of the system and not the ruler of the system.

If X equals humans in this left brain extreme and thus makes them only able to see parts and Y equals other life forms not in this left extreme and thus able to see things in as a whole then X will always dominate the Y's because X only sees itself as important.

$X + Y = -Y$ or $+X$

As X increases Y decreases because X only sees itself as important and that means it eliminates any Y's in its way.

X perceives its life is more important and Y see's all life as important so Y is at a disadvantage because it will not even stand against X because it perceives X is as important as itself. X will always destroy or control Y because X only sees itself as important. This throws the equilibrium off. This leads to a situation where there is many X's and nearly no Y's. So an X arrives in a situation where there are many Y's and the Y's see the X as important as they are, but X only sees itself as important and thus only see's other X's as important so eventually X will change the balance to where there are only X's and all the Y's are gone and Y will allow that because Y see's the X's as important as itself .

So in any situation X is always going to win over Y because X only sees itself as important and Y sees X as important also because Y see's wholes and thus finds everything of value. When the Y's are the minority then X is the majority but the X's also fight among their self because when all is said and done the X's see their own self as the most important thing even over other X's. So the X's arrive in an area where there are many Y's and X determines the Y's are not like it so it starts to dominate them. The Y's see the X's as equals so they do not resist. Eventually this means the X's will dominate all the Y's and then the whole system will be dominated by the X's on all levels and what will be left are just X's. Then the X's will try to dominate each other but because each X thinks of itself as most important there will be much conflict and so only the most dominate X's will come to the top and they will control all the X's below them. This will lead the X's who are being controlled to resist because they see their self as most important and this will force the dominate X's to need even greater leverage to keep control over the X's under it. This creates an infinite struggle and ever increasing tension between the X's that dominate over the lower X's it controls. Eventually the X's who are being controlled will revolt over the X's that control it but this will not end the conflict because eventually dominate X's will come to the top and start the cycle all over again. So the X's are extreme left brained because of the education conditioning and this means there will always be conflict even among the X's and when the X's come in contact with the Y's who see things as a whole the X's will dominate them also. This never ending conflict is a symptom the X's only see things as parts so they can never be at peace or in harmony with other X's or Y's. This will eventually lead to the X's destroying their self because a system that has conflict as a foundation cannot last. Only a system of harmony can be sustained which means only the Y's that see things as a whole can be sustained. The X's are even divided among their self so even when everything in sight is an X they will still have conflict. This X state is also in conflict with other X states. So the X state is in conflict with other X states or groups and also is in conflict with itself until the entire system collapses. This means the X's are a threat to the Y's and their self and so they are unviable as an organism and if allowed to continue they will not only destroy their self but the Y's and the entire system. Real life example of this is the X's came to America and saw the Y's, Native Americans, and wiped them out. The X's may argue they did not wipe them out but that is because they are too stupid to understand they did wipe them out and would wipe them out again, and wipe them out again into infinitely. Sie können dieses X-Ygesetz benennen, das ich gerade die Rohrer nie sogar versuchte Theorie verursachte.- 8:41:00 PM

[Exodus 2: 11   And it came to pass in those days, when Moses was grown, that he went out unto his brethren, and looked on their burdens: and he spied an Egyptian smiting an Hebrew, one of his brethren.

12 And he looked this way and that way, and when he saw that there was no man, he slew the Egyptian, and hid him in the sand.

13 And when he went out the second day, behold, two men of the Hebrews strove together: and he said to him that did the wrong, Wherefore smitest thou thy fellow?

14 And he said, Who made thee a prince and a judge over us? intendest thou to kill me, as thou killedst the Egyptian? And Moses feared, and said, Surely this thing is known.

15 Now when Pharaoh heard this thing, he sought to slay Moses. But Moses fled from the face of Pharaoh, and dwelt in the land of Midian: and he sat down by a well.]

This section is simply saying. Moses woke up from the neurosis and started killing the ones in neurosis because they were unviable as an organism and when the powers that be of the ones in neurosis heard of this they decided to kill Moses. So this is when Moses became what would be known today a terrorist and a mass murderer or a person who fights against what is known as civilization. Moses decided to fight against the slave making machine and the taskmaster does not like it when his slaves are in question so they determine to kill any threat to their power and slaves. So after the powers that be, of the ones in neurosis, put a price on Moses' head, Moses fled into the wilderness and joined the tribes of the ones who were not in neurosis and started making his plan for an all out attack on civilization. In (13) two who were not in neurosis asked Moses why he killed the one in neurosis and Moses said, Who made them the judge over other people? Who said they could control people? Who said they could make slaves of everyone? Who said they have a right to make slaves of the ones who do not get the education or do poorly at it? Moses then says, they want to kill me and control me and turn me into a slave when I want to free people from being slaves to these ones in neurosis. Then Moses said surly you know why I killed them, because they are of unsound mind because they are in neurosis and that is all I can do to them because they are going to ruin everything in their path is one does not kill them. Moses was afraid the ones he met did not know that because the ones he met were ones who never got the education and so they did not understand the whole of the problem.

Moses was in the neurosis and in civilization and then he woke up so he was fully aware of what it did to him so he had the contrast of knowing the difference. This is why for example the Incas trusted the Spanish because they did not know who they were dealing with. This is why Native Americans trusted the white man at first because they did not know they were dealing with ones in neurosis until it was too late. This contrast is similar to when a person fights in a war they are not so eager to go to war and when a person does not have that experience they are ignorant to it.

It is like when a person kicks a drugs habit they know what they went through so they have the contrast of the experience. So Moses was in neurosis and got the education and knew what he had to do to himself to get out of the neurosis so he had the contrast and knew how devastating it was and the two he spoke with were never in neurosis so they didn't understand why Moses was so on fire against the ones in neurosis.

In (11) this comment "when Moses was grown" means when Moses woke up from the neurosis which means somehow he applied fear not, perhaps he was meek. Wink wink.

Meek is one who is suicidal because they do not perceive their life is even worth living and that is a symptom of one in neurosis. So the suicidal are suicidal because they are in this extreme left brain state and once in a while one messes up and accidentally breaks the curse or gets out of the extreme left brain state because they come close to dying and then do not try to save their self, which is suicidal, and then they don't die, so they wake up or apply fear not.

"And Moses feared, and said, Surely this thing is known" Moses was concerned these ones not in neurosis and never were in neurosis would understand his actions of killing the ones in neurosis. The deeper meaning of this text is Moses hated what the education did to his mind and so he hated being aware of what it was doing to others so he felt if he wiped out the power structure of the civilization the education would stop and so would the neurosis. This of course is vanity because the strong point of the education is although is veils the right brain it still looks good for 'food" and still appears to make one knowledgeable or wise. One might suggest this education is the perfect drug. The mental effects are absolute and the remedy is nearly impossible to apply intentionally so it is a fatal condition psychology and physiologically on a personal and environmental level. - 9/12/2009 12:48:33 AM

1:22:05 AM – The point about Genesis and Exodus is Moses was not around at the time of Abraham and Isaac. Perhaps Abraham was one of the first to wake up from the neurosis and then record a written record outside of Adam at this location in the world, and that is proof he got the education and thus the neurosis. Adam speaks of the cause of the neurosis which is tree of knowledge and also he speaks of the Egyptians and hieroglyphics going back perhaps as far as 4000 BCE. Abraham may be the most important person in the entire western religion because he clarified what the remedy of the neurosis was, fear not he also gave a good example, Abraham and Isaac method. [Genesis 15:1 After these things the word of the LORD came unto Abram in a vision, saying, Fear not, Abram: I am thy shield, and thy exceeding great reward.]

So Abraham or Abram is the first human being in the west to get the education and the neurosis and then wake up from it and identify a remedy in practical terms. He recorded this in text and that text survived but perhaps others tried but their texts did not survive. Of course the sane never figured out what his texts meant so it perhaps does not matter his texts survived.

So Abram was the first one to document a practical solution to this neurosis in the west and document it and have those documents survive. The reason one can tell Abram lived long before Moses is because Abram did not attempt to reason with the ones in neurosis he simply burned down their cities and killed them out right. Moses tried to reason with them with words and then he still did not burn down their cities so that shows the cities were far too large by the time of Moses.

[Genesis 13:12 Abram dwelled in the land of Canaan, and Lot dwelled in the cities of the plain, and pitched his tent toward Sodom.]

This comment shows Lot was a spy for Abram so Lot and Abram both woke up from the neurosis and decided to destroy these cities and they suggested this because the cities were full of these ones in neurosis and so they could only be eliminated.

[Genesis 13:13   But the men of Sodom were wicked and sinners before the LORD exceedingly.]

This is not suggesting supernatural this is suggesting they got the education and were mentally unsound and thus rabid. The reason Abram wrote was because he got the neurosis. A child is taught to write and they get the neurosis unless they get taught properly and I am uncertain how that would be because written language is sequential based and so anyone not in neurosis could not write. Really there are perhaps only two kinds of people the ones who get the education and are in neurosis and the ones who get the education and break the curse of the neurosis. Relative to the time period of genesis there was people who had the neurosis, people who broke the curse and people who could not write at all.

So Lot and Abraham were what one would consider today as terrorist against civilization and they were far less merciful than Moses was or they had a better chance against civilization than Moses had because the cities were relatively small.

[Genesis 18:20 And the LORD said, Because the cry of Sodom and Gomorrah is great, and because their sin is very grievous;]

The cry was great denotes these cities were rather large but not as large as the cities at the time of Moses so it is difficult to guess exactly when Abraham was around but it certainly was not at a time were cities had large armies to protect them in fact the large armies of the Egyptians in Moses' time were perhaps an answer to the fact the ones not in neurosis were attacking them. They would be considered barbarians and they would attack the cities and so the cities would need standing armies.

[Genesis 18:23 And Abraham drew near, and said, Wilt thou also destroy the righteous with the wicked?]

This comment shows that Abram was explaining there is no point in reasoning with the ones in neurosis. This is similar to Catholic exorcism instructions that one should never reason with a demon. Abram is saying should I just try to reason with them or kill them all and just burn down the cities. Then he says [Genesis 18:26 And the LORD said, If I find in Sodom fifty righteous within the city, then I will spare all the place for their sakes.]

This is indicative of the neurosis. For one, written language and math looks great and so everyone wants to learn it and so anyone who doesn't learn it is at a disadvantage in these cities. This is just like today if a person does not have a high school education they are pretty much unable to survive at all in civilization, so Abram is saying there is not even fifty in this city that do not have the neurosis so burn it all and kill them all.

[Genesis 19:1 And there came two angels to Sodom at even; and Lot sat in the gate of Sodom: and Lot seeing them rose up to meet them; and he bowed himself with his face toward the ground;]

This comment shows Lot was at the gate so he was like a look out or a spy for Abraham. Lot sat at the gate which means he watched the gate so he was a lookout. In today's world it would be looked at as getting intelligence on the enemy. "Rose to meet the angels" is suggesting armies. So there were two groups or "angels" which is saying armies. Lot met them at the gate and turning his eyes to the ground suggested he told them what he knew. He perhaps drew the battle plan in the sand. So he was letting the armies know where the enemies weakness was. This suggestion of angels is similar to how today one in trouble will say "When does the cavalry get here." or "When are they sending the cavalry." So up to this point Lot is spying the cities and then the cavalry arrives and he tells them what he knows.

[Genesis 19:15 And when the morning arose, then the angels hastened Lot, saying, Arise, take thy wife, and thy two daughters, which are here; lest thou be consumed in the iniquity of the city.]

This is Lot being in a situation where he knows they are getting ready to burn this city and his family is in that city and perhaps even under the neurosis. So he is in a harsh situation where he has to convince his family to leave the safety of the city and go back to the wilderness so he has to chose and quickly. The armies, angels, are telling Lot we are getting ready to attack so if you want your family to survive you better get them out now. So this line is a dramatic moment where Lot has to chose between his family and this "mission" he is on.

[Genesis 19:16 And while he lingered, the men laid hold upon his hand, and upon the hand of his wife, and upon the hand of his two daughters; the LORD being merciful unto him: and they brought him forth, and set him without the city.]

This is saying Lot convinced his family to leave the city which is civilization itself.

[Genesis 19:17 And it came to pass, when they had brought them forth abroad, that he said, Escape for thy life; look not behind thee, neither stay thou in all the plain; escape to the mountain, lest thou be consumed.]

Escape to the mountain is saying go back to the wilderness. Most cities were built on flat plains so to the mountains suggest wilderness. This is similar to head for the hills. It's an expression meaning trouble is coming. "Look not behind thee" is relative to once one breaks the neurosis they cannot remember much of what they were like in the neurosis. It is as if one cannot even remember their life in neurosis. So it is saying forget about the city and civilization and also you will forget about how you use to be after the remedy is applied completely. The past mental state will just be like a bad dream but a bad dream one is unable to really relate to. That's not a good description the best way to look at it is after the remedy is applied one within a year cannot remember their past mental state in neurosis because it was so full of emotions and one no longer can relate to that kind of strong emotions so it's like a dream or a past life one vaguely remembers. "Escape for thy life" means get away from this civilization that thrusts this education on people for you mental life's sake.

[Genesis 19:20 Behold now, this city is near to flee unto, and it is a little one: Oh, let me escape thither, (is it not a little one?) and my soul shall live.]

A little city is a village as in a tribal village not a city.

9/14/2009 12:38:33 AM
[Genesis 50:17 So shall ye say unto Joseph, Forgive, I pray thee now, the trespass of thy brethren, and their sin; for they did unto thee evil: and now, we pray thee, forgive the trespass of the servants of the God of thy father. And Joseph wept when they spake unto him.]

This comment relates to forgiveness of the ones who sin. "For they did unto thee evil" means the ones who forced this written education and math on you which made you extreme left brained and then you had to go through this fear not fire to break that curse. Once one breaks the curse they are going to be mentally, fully aware of what happened to them. At times they are going to feel this vengeance temptation. At times they are going to be searching for heads to make up for this mental rape that they understand happened to them. Simply put at times after one breaks the curse they are going to want paybacks. Is est quare is est valde maximus parumper alio reor dilgenter pro adicio is vereor non ut excito sursum ex vomica. Is est non a jugis mens tamen illic ero vicis unus ero insulted per ones quisnam had a manus manus in suum mental rape quod unus mos volo percello lemma.

"I pray thee now, the trespass of thy brethren, and their sin; for they did unto thee evil:"

One should do the best they can to tolerate the evil ones but every person who wakes up has their own agenda or vengeance mission to play out. Saya sudah memutuskan menenggelamkan pelacur jahat itu dengan buku saya dan jika mereka masuk cara saya saya akan membinasakan mereka. pri pameti sam sebe cio biće odmor na tvornica JA odlučio je da pisati beskonačan knjiga. Oni bi trebao moliti za njihovo kurva bog ogledni primjerak JA ne odlučio je da to čepljenje pisanje beskonačan knjiga.

So this comment "And Joseph wept when they spake unto him." Is saying if you apply this fear not you will wake up to the fact you got mentally raped and then you also be aware the sane are still

94

mentally raping children on a daily basis, and then you are suppose to try to do your best to ignore that. Simply put you are going to wake up and be aware of crimes far worse than mass murder and you are expected to look the other way. You will understand the definition of the comment man's inhumanity to man and you will not be able to get any justice ever.

The sane will laugh in your face and then brag about how many children they mentally raped with their education because they do not apply fear not to the children and then you will not be able to do anything or they will call you a threat. One is perhaps better off not waking up because of this one aspect alone. Reaching nirvana or enlightenment or achieving mental harmony sounds like a great idea and is, but one is going to lose all their ignorance and drugs are not going to ease ones mental gnashing of teeth from the loss of ignorance. So "And Joseph wept" means Joseph was gnashing his teeth because he was aware of what sane do and have done and will continue to do, and Joseph is being asked to forgive them for they know not what they do. The sane may not be able to grasp what I am saying but the ones who are awake understand fully what I am saying. - 1:05:18 AM

3:18:06 AM – [Genesis 37:23 And it came to pass, when Joseph was come unto his brethren, that they stript Joseph out of his coat, his coat of many colours that was on him;

Genesis 37:28 Then there passed by Midianites merchantmen; and they drew and lifted up Joseph out of the pit, and sold Joseph to the Ishmeelites for twenty pieces of silver: and they brought Joseph into Egypt.]

Stripped Joseph of his many colors denotes he was robbed of his mind. He was robbed of his right brain. He was sold for twenty silver means he was robbed of his mind for money. This is similar to how many are robbed of their mind with the promise of money. "You get an education so you will make lots of money." The catch is those years of left brain written language and math are going to leave you so far into left brain and thus veil your right brain ,all the money in the universe is not going to bring your mind back.

Brought Joseph to Egypt denotes he was brought into civilization or civilization is the ones who force the education on people and then do not suggest the fear not remedy so they leave people with a mentally unsound mind and rob them of their colors which is right brain.

This education totally kills a person mentally so it is a crime far beyond the realms of murder and rape and molestation because its destroys a person's potential for their entire life in 99% of the cases. Simply put there is no worse crime in the universe. The worse thing about is that the people who get the education get it at such a young age they never get to experience what it is like to have a sound mind so they are robbed of their life all together. One simply is mentally dead after the years of left brain education so they are mentally dead yet they perceive they are not mentally dead so they are also blind to the fact they are mentally dead.

4:45:10 PM – Antisocial personality disorder is essentially a person who disregards the rights and well being of others. This appears to be a person who hurts others and then is aware of it but in reality it is a person who does things that in fact harm others but they are not aware that is what it is doing. A person who dumps oil in a river to save money for disposal knows what they are doing but they simply can live with it or the consequences do not bother them.

A person who abuses a child and knows they are is simply a person who is not concerned about others rights but is none the less aware of what they are doing. So then it comes to a person who is harming others and they are not aware they are. That is traditionally what is known as an insane person. An insane person can go harm many people but never mentally be aware they are so they very unstable because they harm others but do not think they are harming others so they continue to do it. So this type of insane person perceives what they do is right or proper when in reality they are harming people so they are very mentally unstable because they do not know what they do.

A bad person for example may go out and harm people and that is their main goal. They understand what they are doing so no matter what they do they are not insane. In contrast the insane type person can harm thousands of people yet still sleep perfectly at night and even believe they are righteous in their deeds even when in reality their deeds are harmful; to their self and to ones around them. The point of this is all of society in general supports this written education and math. In reality after one teaches this education it veils right brain and thus harms that person who gets the education, yet all of society keeps doing this to the next generation and also had the education done to their self, and they all believe they are righteous for continuing to do it.

The teachers are harming children because they do not understand the consequences of what this education does to the mind if the fear not conditioning is not applied. The school system itself is not aware of the consequences. The government itself is not aware of the consequences. The people who vote to make the government and teachers and school system keep using this education without any suggestion of the consequences or the remedy to counter act this left brain conditioning are all text book examples of antisocial insane people.

None of these people are aware of what every action has an equal and opposite reaction means. They believe if you make a person do many years of left brain sequential conditioning that person will not end up with an unsound mind. These people believe after many years of left brain intensive conditioning a person will in fact end up wise or with a sound mind. These people simply cannot grasp what cause and effect means and that is a symptom they have been conditioned to extreme left brain and so their mind is only able to have sequential thoughts so they cannot understand what this left brain intensive conditioning does to others because they would have to admit they got it also and it has ruined them mentally as a result.

These people are unable to grasp that when they do not eat for one day and then they feel weak and hungry it is not a symptom they need to eat it is a symptom their mind is so unbalanced it is telling them things that are not true. One should not be hungry and thus weak and irritable and slothful after one day without food but these people can seldom go six hours without eating because they do start to get weak and slothful and irritable.

A person who is hallucinating on this level cannot be anything but a danger to everyone around them and their self but they do not perceive they are a danger to their self or others. They are eating way too much food for example and it is killing them and they do not think it is. They are nervous wrecks and have way too many emotions but they do not think they do. They cannot think clearly and because they got the education at such a young age they cannot even tell what thinking clearly even is. These people have no contrast. Their colors where ripped from them when they were so young, their mind, they never got to feel what a sound mind is like. They see these wise ones down through history and they think "Why aren't I as smart as Einstein or Edison or Tesla?". They think that their genes are bad or their mind is not as smart because they cannot grasp that in reality their mind is so unsound from all these years of left brain conditioning it is not even functioning much anymore in contrast to a sound mind.

These people take all kinds of drugs as recreation and as relaxation drugs and they perceives the drugs are working on them and making them euphoric but in reality the drugs are silencing that left brain for a little while and they are feeling the power of the right brain so they are not high at all they are getting a slight taste of what it feels like when one is of sound mind.

They want that feeling so they keep taking drugs but the drugs will kill them or harm them so they are proper to want to feel right brain because it is theirs but they go about it the wrong way so they end up harming their self. This is a symptom of being unable to think clearly. They all have a bottleneck. The bottle neck is that they are mentally so far to the left they cannot make any complex thoughts because complexity is right brain so they make sequential deductions. "Take drugs feel good." The ones who do not take any drugs after they get the education are worse off than the ones who do because they have settled in their mind on the fact they will never amount to much. They have given up on their mind. The ones who do the drugs after the education are at least trying to break out of the extreme left brain state of mind, they are looking for an awakening as it were.

They are aware something is wrong and so they are using drugs to experiment and try to break out of this mental jail cell they are in but they are trapped because the bottleneck will not allow them to think clearly to break out. They are under the influence of the left brains sequential thoughts and so they spend their whole life trying to get out of that state of mind because they are aware something is wrong but their efforts usually ends up killing them because their thoughts are sequential and thus they go very slowly.

The complexity here is once one applies the fear conditioning and breaks out of the left brain state of mind they no longer desire drugs or are even able to feel euphoria from the drugs, so the only people who do drugs for the euphoria are people still in the left brain extreme state of mind caused by the many years of education which is simply left brain conditioning to an extreme. But of course the ones in this extreme left brain state of mind cannot grasp that because their thoughts are not complex enough to understand that. All of these things are elementary to ones of sound mind but to ones of unsound mind or in extreme left brain they are simply too complex for them to ever grasp.

It is not the ones in neurosis are stupid it is simply they got so much left brain conditioning their minds are unsound on every level one can imagine and they need drugs just to feel slightly normal again. It takes major drugs just for them to feel good. It takes major drugs just for them to feel less nervous for a moment. It takes major drugs just for them to think clearly for a moment. It takes major drugs just for them to be creative for a moment. The problem is drugs costs money and are not a permanent solution so their desire to feel good is proper but the way they go about it cannot be maintained. This does not mean they are losers this means they were mentally abused by adults that had no business conditioning a child at such a young age into such an extreme left brain state to begin with. So the adults are to blame because they have no business being around children when all they do is mentally rape them because they are in extreme left brain state and perceive they help children when in reality they mentally ruin children because they cannot mentally understand what the result of all this left brain sequential education is going to do to a child that does not even have a fully developed mind. If they do not apply the counter remedy to the left brain conditioning which is a fear conditioning aspect they ruin the child's mind and thus ruin the child.

The greatest logic these left brain adults can come up with is the child is stupid because it cannot pass all of these left brain tests when in reality a child who does not do well at all the left brain tests, it is simply a child who is not taking the mental damage as easily as other children do. So these children who do not "make the grade" are considered dumb and thus become outcasts and are given slave jobs when in reality the left brain conditioning just didn't take to well for them. Some human beings do not take well to being mentally raped and some under the right threats of punishment or abuse take to it well. "If you do not get better grades this semester you will be punished" is simply a scare tactic to make the child destroy their own mind. Mi capita spesso riflettere perché consentono di sano anche il mio respiro ossigeno.

The child is in a position where they trust the adults and so they assume the adults would never harm them and so when an adult threatens them with punishment they try as hard as they can to force this sequential mind damaging conditioning on their self so they will not be beaten by their parents. This is why all bets are off in the war. As regras do estupradores mental não se aplica a mim.

"And they believe rightly; for I have sworn upon the altar of god, eternal hostility against every form of tyranny over the mind of man. But this is all they have to fear from me"

Thomas Jefferson

Jestliže jeden je násilník mentální, duševní smrt je vše, co je, a všichni chápou, tak nepřátelství je jediný způsob, jak komunikovat s ním.- 5:45:39 PM

7:39:12 PM – Society creates all these laws that are simply methods to punish people that exhibit these symptoms that are a result of the extreme left brain education conditioning because society does not have the intelligence to understand what this left brain conditioning does to a person. So society creates the mental problems initially by forcing this left brain education on children, then does not have the intelligence to use the counter remedy which is fear conditioning so it does not leave the child in mental hell. Then society makes money off of the people it conditions by creating laws so it can put these people it damaged in cages. This is simply an elementary profit or slave machine technique. Create the problem and then make money off of that problem. This is relevant to so many levels. The pharmaceutical company makes profit from making psychological drugs and drugs that cure all these physical ailments caused by the extreme left brain conditioning: Depression, Stress, High Blood pressure, Ulcers, Obesity, a host of emotional problems, and infinite others.

The powers that be find it easy to control people who are prone to fear and are basically mentally hindered to the point of retardation. It's very easy to take advantage of a human that has mental retardation but it is very difficult to control a human being of sound mind and thus one that is not prone to fear. "Get in your cage and fall in line or fearful things will happen to you." That is what society is. "You will die without our help."

People believe these tactics because they have no faith in their own mind because society raped their mind when they were a child. They never had brain function so they perceive their 10% brain function is normal brain function. They are too mentally hindered to understand what normal brain function is and society has made sure of that by this forced education under the guise of wisdom and under the force of law.

An adult will be thrown in jail if they do not educate their child with the left brain conditioning. There is no freedom, "You condition your child with our left brain conditioning factories or you go to jail and we will tell everyone you hate your child." - 7:51:46 PM

9/14/2009 11:47:45 PM – The most difficult part of understanding this neurosis is to first understand there is two hemispheres of the brain and then understanding left brain is sequential based or good at sequential aspects and right brain is good at random access aspects. People who understand the brain have no problem understanding that, but people who do not may not even be aware of that. So that's the first important concept to be aware of. After one understands those traits of the mind then the possibility that education does in fact condition one to left brain is more believable.

One thing a person who has been conditioned has the most difficulty with is doubt or ambiguity because that is a right brain trait and so that aspect of the mind is veiled so they have trouble doubting. They have trouble doubting these many years of sequential education perhaps did condition them into left brain. They will perhaps say that is not even possible but that is because they are unable to doubt or question. What they have trouble thinking is maybe all those years of left brain education did condition them into an unsound state of mind.

The next part is to understand what classes in school besides written language, reading and math are sequential based classes. For example history class, history is sequential based because one has to keep all these dates in sequential order in their mind. What happened first and then next. History is sequential based so that class is all about sequence and then one has to write about it using a language that is sequence based.

Next there is physical education. Counting is all about physical education. How many sit ups can you do in 60 seconds. How many laps did you run? Who is winning the game. How many points did you win by? What are the rules of the game? Even though it is subtle one's mind is thinking in sequence and thinking about rules.

Economics is all about numbers again. Counting numbers and keeping numbers in sequence, finding out differences in various numbers. The thing about all of these is it puts this sequencing in the mind. When one is adding numbers in their mind they are really sequencing. When one is thinking about what they are going to say they are thinking about how to arrange the sentence they are going to say in proper sequence.

Home economics is about rules. What one should do and what one should not do. Then in home economics there is cooking. Cooking has a recipe and that recipe is in sequence. First you add this ingredient then you add this ingredient.

Music class is based on musical notes and they are based on the alphabet that is in sequence. The musical arrangement is labeled by measures and each measure has a number and each composition has a certain amount of measures. Counting off the beats for a composition is also in sequence. One, two, three, four. While a musician is playing a composition they have this count going on in their head. That counting is in fact left brain conditioning. Everyone time a person thinks about these sequences in writing, reading or math they are conditioning into left brain.

On top of that there are rules to all of this sequencing and that is also a left brain trait.

Then there is the one class in all of school that may be considered right brain and that is art class. The irony there is anyone who takes art class is looked at as stupid or dumb. On top of that there are rules to what you can and cannot draw in art class. One cannot draw a picture freely they are constantly thinking "If I draw that picture will they send me to the psychologist office for a mental evaluation?" So this again is an example of these rules that are going on in a person's mind at all times, these unspoken rules that a person is conditioned to adhere to in fact condition them further into left brain. Right brain hates rules because right brain is so complex and rules hinder complexity. One cannot think out of the box or be open minded if they have all these rules to follow because rules inhibit creativity and complexity.

So school itself is completely left brain driven. Simply put, written language, reading and math are the cornerstones for all the other classes. One cannot do the history if they cannot read and count. One cannot do the music if they cannot read and count. One cannot do the economics if they cannot read and count. The problem is what kind of class would there be that is based on random access thoughts and no rules. The answer is none. No rules goes against the grain of society itself.

To one conditioned to left brain no rules is a nightmare. They see people running wild killing each other when they hear no rules because they are so far into left brain and left brain loves rules and makes a person think the more rules they have the safer they are. The conditioning is so absolute everything is a symptom of it.

Once one is conditioned to left brain their sequential logic will not allow them to see things properly. The sequential thoughts hinder their ability to see the whole picture so they are in this cage mentally and they can hardly see past the bars. This tree of knowledge which is known as school is based on the three R's and the three R's are sequential based. So this means if one wants to three R's which is pretty much a given, and one also wants a sound mind, they are going to have to go through the fire which is apply fear not and that is mental suicide. This is what cause and effect is all about here.

If one wants the knowledge tree they are going to have to kill their self mentally in order to keep their mind or keep a sound mind. One has to pay the piper for this knowledge or they end up mentally dead. I am not talking about aliens or ghosts here I am talking about obvious effects from an obvious cause. If one gets the drug they are going to have to do some very harsh things to counter act the drug. This is why the tree of knowledge does not make one wise it gives one this burden around their neck because once they are conditioned they are going to have to do something to counter that conditioning and that is face their own fear of death, and do not run from it, and that is perhaps not worth the knowledge to begin with.

If one does not want to apply the remedy after they get the conditioning that is fine but they are going to be mentally unsound and mentally as abnormal as one can ever be. All the narcotics in the universe will not mentally mess a person up more than all these years of left brain conditioning do. Drugs law are to protect the children from brain damage and education mentally damages the children and in turn cause the children to want to do drugs.

One has this language in their head but once they condition away the fear they will no longer be able to use the language that appears proper to the ones still conditioned. One will lose their ability to sequence sentences properly relative to the norms of the ones conditioned into extreme left brain. One will lose their ability to use commas properly. This is all because they will see things as a whole and they will get the spirit of the sentences they write and they will no longer be looking just for parts like each word, and detecting parts is left brain.

So one will appear on drugs or dumb or stupid to ones conditioned into extreme left brain that have no applied the remedy. These poorly disguised diaries appear right to me but if an English major graded them I perhaps would not get more than a page or two of proper sentences, based on the "rules" of language so I would be deemed stupid. This is a harsh reality for some who were never aware of this to fully grasp but the truth is, when one has silenced emotions after applying the remedy they simply accept it as an observation and not an emotional situation. - 12:53:32 AM

12:59:12 AM – I am an accident and I know nothing of these other methods such as meditate in your safe home at night. I look at what I experienced as an Abraham and Isaac, or a "those who lose their life(mentally) will preserve it" or a "submit to fear of perceived death" or a sit in a cemetery and face your fear of perceived death and allow it, on a mental level of course. Defeat death.

The thing is, one may negate this left brain conditioning to a degree but unless they go the full measure and defeat their fear of perceived death one may end up trapped somewhere up the hill so to speak. Perhaps no one on the left understands what I say anyway so there is no point in beating round the bush, so to speak. - 1:03:41 AM

If one wants to be a part of the solution and assist others properly, it is best they mentally let go of their self first.

4:01:58 AM – Once the right brain is veiled from the education complexity and creativity is veiled and on a species level that means the species has trouble making complex decisions. The species cannot handle complex problems so it makes some missteps. Over population is a misstep. Destroying the environment is a misstep.

Going to war with each other is a misstep. Looking at the species as all these separate parts or countries is a misstep. A country only see's itself so its world stops at its borders. That's a misstep because it creates this false sense of measure in relation to the world. One country looks at the population of another country and determines it needs to build its population up so it is not outnumbered by the second country.

What this all leads to is battles of population and thus overpopulation on a world scale. This is a symptom of the left brain making a person think they are most important. This is what is known as a God complex and it can be taken out to each country thinking it is more important than the other countries, and thus their world view or the whole species view is ignored.

So there are all these countries and each country is competing in population against countries near it with no regards to the world population. It is a "me first" attitude. This is a symptom of being in extreme left brain and only seeing things as parts. This goes right back to the education where a child is graded on how well they spell words and a word is letters and thus parts.

So a child is graded on how well they arrange those letters or part's so then a child grows up and only sees parts. National identity means parts. State identity means parts. This leads to the conflicts because then one who only sees parts and starts suggesting their country or state is better than another country or state and that is not possible because all the countries have people in them. So this is what the god complex is. My country is better than yours. My race is better than yours. My ideals are better than yours and then within the country there are all these parts again. My religion is better than yours. My political view is better than yours. All these conflicts start coming to the surface because the people only see things as parts.

They are really just labels and they are expected when a person is in extreme left brain so they are not something that can be addressed because to the people in extreme left brain they seems like normal judgments. Simply put these labels and judgments seem logical to a person in extreme left brain but they are in fact not logical because we are one species.

This all goes back to making many missteps because the complexity and creativity of right brain is veiled. The random access processing of right brain is veiled so as a whole the species cannot see very far in front of its nose. The species tries to make a long term decision but it cannot make a proper long term decision it can only make short term decisions. One cannot make a long term decision because sequential thought will not allow complexity in that decision. It gives off the impression everything is s surprise because one cannot see very far down the road because the sequential thoughts will not allow it. So the education itself is good and in fact very good but the remedy to keep one's mind sound and in harmony is equally harsh. So this demotic and math has certainly dug us into a hole. We cannot get rid of written language and math so we will keep conditioning the next generation into this unsound extreme left brain and we will keep making missteps and eventually we will commit suicide as a species.

Perhaps the sane cannot see that far down the road to understand that is the logical conclusion. Nature will not allow a creature with a defect to survive. Somehow nature is this harmony thing and when some creature has as defect it gets out of harmony and that disharmony is nature's way of eliminating that defective creature. Only the strong or sound creatures survive and the rest are defeated by their disharmony.

As a species we have done some major damage to ourselves and the environment in the last five thousand years yet we understand we have been around for perhaps 200,000 years. This is an indication how fast we are destroying our only means of survival. The whole species is essentially only looking at parts and so a species that is in conflict with itself will destroy itself. This is a symptom of what nature is doing to get rid of this defective creature.

We have inadvertently made ourselves defective or out of harmony and nature does not play games or favorites. Nature will wipe us all out one way or another because we are way out of harmony and nature will not shed one tear. Nature is harmony and we are out of harmony and nature always wins. Perhaps the sane do not see that. Perhaps the sane perceive all these emotional problem and wars and physiological ailments and conflicts on every scale are simply natural but they are not natural they are a symptom the species is coming apart.

One can silence the right brain of any creature and it will not be viable. Nature gave us two hemispheres for a reason and if we inadvertently silence one of those we are not viable. A creature that needs four legs but is born with two is not going to last long. A creature that needs two eyes and is born with no eyes is not going to last long. A fish born without a tail is not going to last long. A bird born without wings is not going to last long. We are born with two hemispheres in working order and after the education one is veiled so the game is over right around 8th grade. Right around 8th grade is when that right brain is pretty much veiled for life unless one goes through the fire so to speak.

That's when the kids start getting depressed and doing drugs and start showing symptoms of this unsound mind state. It starts even young than that but at around 8th grade it is pretty much set in stone and the remedy to the full measure is required. The sane will suggest this person made lots of money so they are just fine mentally and that's shows what the scale of success is for them. The sane tend to think on these strange scales of worth. The sane will destroy entire forests and build a subdivision that no one lives in and then call that success. The sane will build a high rise to heaven and no one will live in it and they will call that success. The sane cannot grasp perhaps there is no other planet we are going to be able to get to before the disharmony does us in.

Abraham and Lot did not burn down those cities because they didn't like them it was because they were aware fully what this strange acting human who got the conditioning would end up doing. Moses only had to see these strange acting humans claiming all the natural resources as their own property to understand what would happen eventually. That's called coveting and that is a symptom of left brain and is really just control. Controlling everything is left brain. Loving someone to death is left brain. Loving something to much is left brain. A person in this extreme left brain loves things so much it harms them and ends up being a weakness. We tend to love ourselves so much we kill off other species and thus seal our own fate.

We have this impossible appetite because of the neurosis and so we tend to destroy other species because we simply are gluttonous. Our species is a hog. We kill everything in our path because we are not aware that's a symptom we mentally are way out of bounds. I do not see a solution to this problem because we keep conditioning the next generation and the remedy is so harsh few will ever wake up fully. The ones who wake up are still damaged. There only ones who are not damaged are the ones who never get the education and they are tiny tribes that live in the Amazon and the whole world thinks they are retarded. There are some who understand this education written language problem and attempt to educate their children with speech instead of written language but it all comes down to the fact their small efforts cannot counter the worlds massive left brain conditioning that it continues to instill.

The bottom line to this is, as a species we should be a lot closer to how the Native Americans lived about 300 years ago than how we are now. How we are now is not a symptom of how much we have progressed, it is a symptom of how much we have digressed. The sane will always come back to their god complex. The sane will suggest we have all these cures now and live longer but the truth is we are not all suppose to be living so long. The sane cannot let go. It all goes back to this unsound mind the education creates in a human being. Every symptom goes back to that extreme left brain state. This sequential state of mind makes one slow or slothful to understand and slothful in their living and slothful in their ability to let go. I would not be aware of how it is going to end up, if it was not going to end up that way. Perhaps the sane cannot understand that. Perhaps I need to pray harder for ignorance. I am far too stupid to lie to you.- 5:15:41 AM

1:31:26 PM – So now we have our knowledge. Now you know we accidentally doomed our self as a species with our great knowledge invention. We couldn't just be we had to try to improve everything and now we have knowledge. We know our children are killing their self because they get bad grades and they are shy and embarrassed. We know we kill each other over grains of dirt and resources. We kill each other over stupid misunderstandings. We all hate each other and we don't even trust other countries or our own country. We hate everything and judge everything and cannot tolerate anything. We hate ourselves and we cannot even tell we do. That's all we know now. I finally understood my vanity is beyond my own understanding, - 1:52:49 PM

2:11:24 PM – The mind is very delicate. Drugs certainly can alter the mind but usually only temporarily. This extreme left brain education not only permanently alters the mind but it alters the mind before the mind can fully develop. The mind is in a perfect state when a person is born but then shortly after this extreme left brain sequential conditioning starts and it is far more damaging than any drug will ever be to the mind.

One can take 20 people who have been conditioned and drop them off in the middle of a jungle and they will not be able to function. They will not be able to live in harmony and they will not be able to adapt because they have been conditioned to such a degree they have lost the ability to use the full spectrum of their mind which is required for a human being to survive. This group of 20 will never be able to satisfy their extreme hunger and extreme thirst and they will become weak and they will not be able to get the food they need because they have been conditioned out of being what they are, mammals.

The tribes in the Amazon have no luxuries but they survive and have survived for thousands of years and they are proof that human beings who have been conditioned are some sort of non human or non mammal. The ones who have been conditioned mock the ones in the Amazon which proves the ones who have been conditioned in fact hate normal human beings. The human beings that have been conditioned cannot mentally ever compare to the intelligence required to live like the tribes do in the Amazon, with no luxuries or medicines or safety nets. All of these luxuries in society are really just safety nets to make up for the fact these ones who have been conditioned can no longer survive on their own. They are simply nonviable creatures, They have to be in cages so they can be taken care of and so they do not harm their self. There are only a hand full of viable humans beings left on this planet and they will soon be wiped out by the sane and I am unable to convince anyone of that. I

110

am certain the sane cannot wait to teach them written language and math and "fix" them. "These tribes are so horrible because they can live in harmony and do not destroy everything in their path." There is only one hell and we are in it. I am not out of hell I just woke up to the fact I am in it. - 2:25:35 PM

Unë mund të ju wake up por tuaj të parë duhet ta kuptoni pse ju jeni në gjumë.

3:06:31 PM – In Yaeda, Tanzania there is one of the few remaining hunter gatherer tribes on the planet..They have been around for 50000 years. They have been labeled as the Hadzabe tribe. There are only about 1500 members left. The land they have lived on for thousands of years is going to be taken from them so the sane will have a nice safari land to hunt animals on for fun. This is exactly what happened to the Native Americans and all the other tribes in the world when they came in contact with the sane.

The sane just take everything in their path and they have the numbers and weapons on their side and they have their delusional laws that make them seem like they are in the right to do so. The tribes never have great numbers because they are mentally sound and understand they cannot just overpopulate and remain viable. So then the sane arrive and see this tribe and understand they can push them around because the tribe is few in number. Of course the nature of the sane is to destroy everything in its path including itself. There is no such thing as harmony in the world of the sane it is all disharmony. Their mind is out of harmony and so their deeds and fruits are out of harmony. It is one in the same. Simply put once the mind is altered by the education the game is over. The sane are defeated by life because of this left brain education before they are even twelve. Everything after that age is simply vanity. All the sane have ever invented are methods to wipe out everything in their path including their self. The sane have invented nothing of value. All of the inventions of the sane are simply remedies to the problems the left brain education causes so they have not done anything but try to put a band aid on a cut they have inflicted that never stops bleeding, so they are vanity. - 3:17:37 PM

111

9/16/2009 10:37:46 AM – Past is past. That's a magical comment because it means everything I have said up to this point is negated and I get try to try again. I get to try to approach this problem again with the understanding I am going to end right back where I started. This whole problem comes down to one comment. It is such a deep comment the sane can never grasp it because this single comment shatters the mind of the sane.

[Genesis 2:17 But of the tree of the knowledge of good and evil, thou shalt not eat of it: for in the day that thou eatest thereof thou shalt surely die.]

This comment means never use the tree of knowledge. That's the only viable solution. If you get the education you mentally die. The sane will never ever be able to understand that because they love the tree of knowledge because they already believe without it they are stupid. All the people running around shooting their mouth off about their vast understanding of these ancient texts should simply never speak of these texts again. Le voy a recordar si alguna vez comprender una frase estos antiguos textos sugieren. The moment one starts playing with this sequential based invention they start altering their mind and all the pills and prayers and kind comments are never going to change that absolute fact. The complex thing about all of this is the tribes who never got the education do not understand the remedy because they never needed to apply it. Only the ones who get the education once in a while break the curse of the extreme left brain curse understand the remedy. They know what it's like, they have the contrast. These beings we known as the wise beings of recorded history had this vengeance to make sure they told everyone what this curse does to a person. Of course the sane never figured out what these wise being were saying because they cannot grasp mentally something so complex but even deeper something, so obvious and so devastating. The sane will speak of truth and justice and I spit in their face because their truth is lies and their justice is rape.

There would have to be school that on one hand teaches language verbally and then does not use the written aspect of language until much further into a child's education. Then it does not grade a child on spelling and does not grade a child on sentence structure. That alone would negate school. That is how difficult this problem is. Every money making profession on the planet is based on how much education one gets. One is left with either get the education or get a slave job. Mentally ruin your mind for money or be an outcast in society.

There is no way to go back and live in the wild because just like in a zoo once they have an animal conditioned to the cage they cannot return it to the wild because it cannot exist in the wild any longer. That's what we are now. We have been conditioned to the cage and so we simply cannot survive in the wild any longer. This is why we can never go back. It is not that we can't go back it is that we are unable to go back. Simply put if we tried to live as normal human beings live we would not be able to do it, so we are left to our cage existence because that is our only choice now. So we are slaves now because slavery is the only possibility for us now.

The sane sit in their little cages and fear going outside in their cities. They hate the crime and the drug addiction and then they tell their self, "This is a good existence." The sane hate their Sodom and Gomorrah and they will kill everything in their path to build bigger cities. The sane see nature as evil so they build these artificial ecological systems called cities to take the place of nature because they fear nature because they can no longer survive in nature, because their minds are so unsound they have been robbed of their complexity and creativity aspect of right brain which is required to live in nature.

One cannot survive when they see nature as evil because nature is the only sound ecological system that is viable for existence. A city is not nature it is an attempt by a mentally unsound creature to make up for its fear of nature and its inability to survive in nature. The sane have wiped out nature to replace it with the artificial ecosystem. The sane have to rely on farms to create food because first off they eat like pigs and secondly they have wiped out all the natural food sources so they have painted their self into a corner. The sane have to have these farms that create their food because there is no way to get the food from nature because nature has been wiped out and the sane will suggest that is progress, because they hate nature. The sane cannot see the top of the pit they are in because the complex aspect of their mind is veiled.

The sane see the darkness in the pit they are in as light. The depressed do not know exactly why they isolate their self in their cage and do not like society but they are aware mentally something is very wrong. The depressed and suicidal among the sane are the only ones who have a chance because at least they are not so mentally blind they see civilization as something that can't get any better. The suicidal and depressed among the sane just want to get out. They are not exactly certain why they want to get out but all they can say is they want to get out, they are ready to get out, they have had enough and simply want to get out. They are aware of where they are at and they just want to get the hell out. They are the meek. The meek at least admit something is wrong unlike the sane who suggest light in the pitch black pit they live in.

What are going to do when you wake up and see the herd running towards the cliff and understand you are unable to stop it? You are going to turn to stone emotionally or to salt emotionally because if you do not the gnashing of teeth will be too great of a burden for your mind to handle. Now I am trying to talk you out of waking up. I do not want you to be aware of what I am aware of and I do not want to be aware of it either. My prayers for ignorance are never answered. Maybe your prayers are answered because all you ask for is money. You pray for your health and are not aware you pray you remain cursed. [Luke 17:33 Whosoever shall seek to save his life shall lose it;.]. Perhaps that one is simply far beyond your understanding. So to clarify, if you pray you pray for poverty and a near death experience and maybe you will get lucky, then after you break the curse you pray for ignorance with the understanding the prayer for ignorance will never be answered. - 11:22:37 AM

12:03:17 PM –
You Blink - http://www.youtube.com/watch?v=zorvbHbwNTQ
Neutral - http://www.youtube.com/watch?v=cHsMnyRrVoI

The songs I add to these poorly disguised diaries are for many reasons. They are for contrast on one hand. If one hates the diaries they will like the music. If one hates the music they will like the diaries. If one hates a song that means they should listen to that song until they like it then they should listen to it until they are indifferent to it. This is self control, which is doing something that left brain suggests you shouldn't do and that in turn starts to silence that extremely dominate left brain and in turn, turns up the veiled right brain.

After the sequential conditioning the mind is like a set of scales that are way out of balance so as one side moves the other side moves also. On the scale of the sane these songs all are horrible but the point is one should mentally be indifferent to sounds. A sound mind should not hate or like sounds they should be indifferent to sounds. It is quite vain to dislike a sound or love a sound because a sound is not even tangible. It is also quite vain to copyright a sound and then charge money for it.

A bird does not charge money for its sounds and that is because it is not engaged in vanity. One who is awake to a degree is forced to follow all of these vain laws so they do not get thrown in jail by the sane. They are forced to subscribe to money and forced to do all of these vain things the sane do because if they do not they will be deemed outcasts and then be demonized by the sane. The sane have the numbers so they have so many minions and these minions are going to force their cult leader's wishes on anyone who does not fall into line.

If one does not subscribe to the vanity of the sane then they are certainly a criminal. The taskmaster has many slaves who carry out his wishes without question and without thinking. The taskmaster's slaves suggest anyone who cannot spell well is stupid and the slaves never question that logic. Certainly if one cannot spell well and use commas well it is absolute proof beyond all reality they are retarded and stupid and worthless. Certainly that kind of logic cannot have any flaws. The minions of the taskmaster have no eyes. You can't trust the dust.

Vanity - http://www.youtube.com/watch?v=4nIhvhnW1lI

They believe their silly needs.
They believe their silly deeds.
They deceive their silly needs.
I won't leave their silly deeds.
They retrieve.
I won't leave.
They aren't very smart.
They didn't get a good start.
They will rip out your heart, their deeds.
They aren't very smart, their silly needs.
They aren't very wise, their silly deeds.
They love their little lies.
They only have small eyes. They have no eyes.
They only have small eyes. They have no eyes.

Apparently I need all the filler I can get. - 12:28:28 PM

12:43:04 PM – In the east there is something called the four noble truths. All these comments are saying is life is suffering and it is possible to be free of that suffering and the technique is meditation. This of course is way out of context and also geared to the ones who got the education and have not broken that extreme left brain curse yet.

The ones who have broken it are no longer suffering mentally because they are of sound mind but to go further they are in neutral mentally. One in extreme left brain tries to have fun or be happy but that is because they are not having fun and are not happy.

One goes on vacation because they perceive they need to relax because they perceive they are not relaxed. One takes drugs to escape because they perceive they need to escape. One needs money to be happy because they perceive they are not happy without money. One needs nice clothes to be happy because they perceive they are not happy without money. All of this is symptom their mind is unsound because if their mind was sound they would have so much cerebral wealth they would not care about all of these materialistic goals to try to become happy.

This materialistic satisfaction desire is not the problem is a symptom one is too far into left brain. Money is not bad but if one who is of unsound mind will harm others in any way to get it so they will think they are happy.

A sound mind is a mind that is not suffering because it is indifferent to all of these desires and craving for material things, so one can feel satisfied. The entire economic system of the sane is based on satisfying these material desires the ones they have conditioned into extreme left brain with the education need filled. This all comes back to the one point that the mind is delicate and if it becomes unbalanced there are major fruits or symptoms that one is going to exhibit.

The final truth of these four truths is meditation but that is very complex. One thing is one who is in extreme left brain has very little patience so they do not want to mediate. The second thing is the mediation is a slow route and one risks getting stuck on their way up the mountain. The third point is, one has to mediate on death or their own death or impermanence and in the west that is a person who is depressed or suicidal so people would recommend that person take their pill to "fix it" if they suggest that is what they doing.

One can fiddle around and play games and try to make a mountain out of mole hill and spend the rest of their sitting around trying to figure out what mediation even is or they can just get it over with in one painless motion which is [Luke 17:33 ; and whosoever shall lose his life shall preserve it.].

This mental suicide is in fact totally painless. It is on a thought level not on a physically painful level. It is a one second decision then it is over and the waking up process begins mentally and that takes about one year to fully wake up.

Mentally at first it is rough maybe the first two months but one has no choice after the remedy is applied to do anything but go with the flow. The right brain once unveiled is going to be doing lots of processing and it is going to be very powerful and so this waking up is a mental shock because one has been asleep.

What one thought was quick when they were asleep, they will find out was sloth. One is going to lose all these thoughts about things they thought were important and they will find out many of the things they use to think were of value are no longer of value. This is why the ones with lots of material wealth are not going to be prone to want to wake up because their mind once awake will no register all that material wealth as valuable any longer.

The sane with millions of dollars will mentally think they are a success but once they wake up their mind will no longer allow them to feel satisfaction from that wealth so they will be neutral and so they will no longer have this "I am wealthy so I am good" mindset. They will come to the realization that all that wealth they chased all their life was vanity and it is of no value any longer and that is a harsh reality to face. They are going to think back about all the things they did to get that wealth and then be aware that wealth no longer has value and so they will see all they did to get that wealth was a great quest of vanity.

Moses killed the sane and so did Abraham and Lot and they burned down their cities and killed many of them and the sane cannot believe that but the even deeper reality is that took so much will power to do on their part. It is a miracle beyond all miracles for one who is awake to kill another person because when they look at them all they see is perfection because of the feeling through vision.

Mohammed didn't want to kill anyone but he knew if this curse kept spreading it would ruin the species so he had to do the one thing that was impossible for him to do. Moses didn't want to kill anyone but he had to try and stop the spread of the curse. Abraham didn't want to burn down those cities and kill those people but he had to try and stop the curse to save us from ourselves. The reality is they failed us. They didn't do enough. They couldn't do enough because it was hurting them to do what they did. One who is awake is docile and not violent and they are surrounded by these violent beasts that would kill them for a few shekel.

The only way the sane could relate to this is for them to think about a person with Ebola. There is no room for mercy or sympathy or compassion because if that person with Ebola gets into the population it is all over. So they isolate this person with that disease

118

and there is no morals or values taken into consideration. So the Native Americans who got to a point of just attacking the "settlers" were demonized because the settlers could never grasp what they represented. The settlers could not grasp they were cursed so they assumed the Native Americans were cursed. The Native Americans were not wiping out all the food sources for a little money the settlers were. One was living in harmony and within their means and one was nothing more than rabidity. - 1:28:00 PM

2:31:30 PM – In relation to this Hadzabe tribe. They communicate using a form of verbal clicking sounds. The big point here is they do not have written language. That's the common denominator in all of these tribes. The sane want to take these peoples land so the sane can have fun killing off wild life vainly. Of course eventually the sane will come up with some reason to destroy them. The sane will invent a law or come up with some form of retarded logic to talk their self into destroying these tribes because the very nature of the sane is destruction of anything that is different than them.

All of recorded history is the same story playing over and over and over. The sane meet the ones without the written language curse and the sane destroy them without mercy. That is all recorded history is. All of the battles between the sane over land and resources is a symptom the sane cannot even get along with their self. The sane cannot tolerate the ones who do not have the curse and cannot tolerate others who do have the curse and that is the curse. This is because the sane are in such an extreme state of left brain they can only see parts. This is what creates the suffering. Suffering caused by suffering which leads to more suffering into infinity. Some might call that hell but I call it reality. - 2:37:26 PM

The fruit of the sane is disharmony so all they reap is abomination. We as a species are just slightly past the point of being able to solve this problem with a pill or a prayer. This problem requires brain function in case anyone in this universe can understand anything I say ever. We need brain function to work our way out of this situation. Does anyone even know what brain function is anymore?

Your prayers and your pills are not brain function in case you are wondering.

For those who like truth why don't you go ask the Hadzabe tribe how many of their children commit suicide when they are 13 or 14 or 15. Why don't you ask them how many people in their tribe are depressed and overweight. Why don't you ask them how many people in their tribe hate life. Why don't you ask them how many people in their tribe are on medications for mental problems. The reason the answer will be none on all of those counts is because they do not have written language so they are not conditioned way too far into left brain.

All these tribes know is they are getting railroaded by the sane. This tribes has lived on that land for thousands of years and then this abomination comes along and decides to take that land from them so it can have a place to hunt so it can have fun. This is why I will never find fault with Abraham, Moses or Mohammed's strategy just to slaughter the lot of them. I find no fault and I never will find fault with that strategy. I find no fault with the Natives Americans strategy to deal with the sane. I find no flaws in that strategy. They did nothing wrong they did the righteous thing. Now I am certain I have blown it. - 3:37:38 PM

There will not be any illusions left.

3:53:24 PM – Because of the complexity of explaining this mental state and given the time period many things were said in these ancient texts that actually complicated the situation. These ancient texts were guides for the ones who broke the curse but when the sane got hold of them they assumed they applied to them.

[Genesis 1:28 And God blessed them, and God said unto them, Be fruitful, and multiply, and replenish the earth, and subdue it: and have dominion over the fish of the sea, and over the fowl of the air, and over every living thing that moveth upon the earth.]

The sane read this an assumed it meant destroy everything in your path, have tons of children with no regard to harmony or longevity or ecology. This was a comment to the ones who broke the curse because their very nature is harmony because they are of sound mind so they do not tend to over populate. The sane have children as a vanity materialistic aspect to show they have worth. The sane assume if they do not have children they are worthless or failures so children are like some sort of sign post of success for the sane so they believe the more they have the wiser they are. The sane believe the entire universe revolves around them and how many children they have. So this comment is trying to suggest to the sound minded that in order to compete against this new form of human that pumps out children with no regards to the consequences we have to multiply to have a chance against them. So this comment later is why this go fourth and multiply comment is made.

[Genesis 6:1 And it came to pass, when men began to multiply on the face of the earth, and daughters were born unto them,]

The men are the ones who got the curse the Lords are the ones who broke the curse. This is saying these men are multiplying like rabbits and what makes that even worse is they are also having women so that means they are going to multiply even faster. This is all relative to the time period because obviously there is no chance to win now. One can write or fight but they will never win against the sane now. Simply put the sane are like the grains of sand in the sea so there is no real fight there are just ones who think there is fight.

The ones who are awake do not mind a defeat because they are mentally in neutral so a win is the same as defeat there is no sorrow or suffering there just is, is. The ones that are awake are in mental infinity so all they have left to do is fight this fight they already know they cannot win and that is okay because defeat does not bother them. One might suggest they have infinite time on their hands and there is nothing else better to do. To the ones who are awake there is nothing else going through their mind but this battle. Everything they say and do is relative to this battle because there is nothing else but this battle.

The strategy they use varies from person to person. Some go around and say they are a spiritual leader or teacher. Some hid behind self help books. Some go to physical war against the sane. They are all at war with the sane but using various techniques. Some also have given up and just try to put it out of their mind but they cannot do that because it is all they really think about. Some gain followings and are okay with money and some detest money and have followings and some detest followings and money, but none of them are wrong they just come up with new approaches to fighting the war with the understanding they can never win in the battle against the sane.

They have infinity job security but not on the scale of the sane. The sane give up in a losing battle and the ones who are awake have been proudly losing for the last at last 2500 years and it never has crossed their mind to give up. A machine never gives up it just processes until it drops. Failure and winning is strictly a concept for the sane. The sane will say "I won that match" and they will feel good about it and then they will say "I lost that match" and they will feel bad about it. The ones who are awake cannot feel in contrast to the sane. The ones who are awake are in neutral mentally so they feel a little bit of everything but nothing for more than a moment. So the true way to describe their mental state is nothingness which means they can experience every emotion but not for long.

This is why they tend to be lone wolfs. A good way to look at this is this relationship between Edison and Tesla. They tried to work together but for various reason it didn't last long. This is the reverse of the sane because the sane love the herd mentality. The sane feel worthless if they are not in a relationship or not in a group, and then if they are not say in a religion or belief system, and then in a country. This is what the herd mentality is and the sane deem anyone who does not subscribe to that herd mentality as mentally unbalanced or antisocial.

The sane can never grasp the reason they like the herd mentality is because they are afraid to be on their own because then they have to think for their self and they cannot do that or have no faith they can do that, so they hang around others and idolize others in hopes the others will think for them.

The sane find someone they deem as smart and then they try to latch onto that person in hopes they will become smart or at least have someone to ask advice from because they have long sense given up on the fact they could think for their self. The truth is they are right, they cannot think for their self because they have been conditioned so far into left brain they are not in the realm of a thinker anymore so they are relegated to the class of a sheep or a follower.

Once one is conditioned so far to the left, life is so hard because one only has the retarded aspect of the brain to think with. Life is hard for them, it is very hard, they are in sorrow because they have this brilliant mind and it is so out of balance they end up with a broken machine that isn't worth anything in contrast to a sound mind.

With a sound mind life is simple with an unsound mind life is a nightmare. Granted they were conditioned into this unbalanced mind by the society they trust, but the important thing is they can get out of it but it is something that is going to cost them what they perceive is normal life. The price they have to mentally pay to get out of this extreme left brain state is a problem because that retarded left brain is going to tell them it's not good or safe or right because left brain is an idiot and its dominate.

The idiot aspect of the mind rules the mind of the sane so they listen to the loudest voice in their head and it's the idiot. It's the false voice but it's the loudest voice so they have to deny the loudest voice to increase the volume of the wise veiled right brain voice. Once they break this curse they will understand they can think their way out of anything and that means they are going to not have self esteem problems and that is bad news for the taskmaster. The taskmaster does not like a person who can stand on a rock. The taskmaster likes his slaves to be bogged down in sand. The taskmaster wants his slaves to rely on him, and a person who can think for their self will not need to rely on the taskmaster any longer.

It all comes down to simple logic. A person is easy to control as long as you keep them sedated. The task master doesn't like any wild horses and my middle name is wild horse. So if you like infinite battles you never can win, we have lots of openings on this team and you get to be the captain and call all the plays all the time, simply because we have lots of ambiguity on this team and we can never tell who may throw the winning touchdown, but we are certain it hasn't been thrown yet.

We have no time for rules because we are too busy losing the infinite battle.

I have at times spoken with ones who are awake to a degree and I ask them, "Why aren't you writing infinite books?" and now I realize I should avoid asking that question because it is an improper question because they cannot write infinite books. I will clarify that one at a later date.- 4:37:49 PM

10:32:12 PM – This comment is another encouragement to the ones who broke the curse to multiply so they would be able to have a chance against the ones who were cursed who multiplied at a great rate,.[Genesis 9:1 And God blessed Noah and his sons, and said unto them, Be fruitful, and multiply, and replenish the earth.]

So "blessed Noah and his son's" means they broke the curse and sons means the ones Noah assisted with breaking the curse using the fear not remedy. Replenish means try to out populate the ones that were still cursed. This of course failed because the ones of sound mind who break the curse are in harmony and it is against their nature to over populate.

Why would someone tell Noah to have children? Because he wasn't having enough children to compete with the cursed ones who breed like rabbits with no regards to the consequences. This is in direct relation to why Native American didn't have huge populations and also why other tribes today do not have huge populations. Huge populations cannot be sustained in a harmonious ecological system. These huge populations are going to make problems by their own merit. Lack of food, lack of space, in fighting are all symptoms of an over populated system.

So the sane read these comments and started populating more and so these comments backfired. These texts were battle plans for ones who broke the curse not for the cursed. The cursed found the battle plans and thought the battle plans were talking about some alien sinister force but certainly not them. All of these ancient texts from the ones in the east to the ones in the west are advice to ones who break the curse not advice to the cursed. They are battle plans against the cursed. Simply put the devil, adversary, antichrist, infidel, sane are the ones who get the education and do not apply the remedy which is fear not or fear conditioning.

I certainly would never write in my own personal diaries the whole world population is essentially the devil, even though I just did. Perhaps you can judge my comma usage up to this point in the diaries and then call me and let me know if I smart or not. - 10:43:44 PM

10:59:28 PM – There is one aspect or concept that is very strange. All of these wise beings wrote with the language and used the language and some wrote more than others. This would give one the impression that once they break the curse if they write too much they will come under the influence of the curse again because they will slowly get sequence education again as they start to learn to write again. I am on the fence about that but if it happens I will just go apply the remedy again.

I am aware I am getting better at spelling again but it's hard for me to judge if I am getting any better at sentence sequencing because it all looks good to me. The commas really are difficult though. I just guess with the commas and paragraphs, this is because I see the sentence as a whole and a comma separates the sentence into parts and is also a judgment call.

One very obvious clue that the tree of knowledge is the written language is the history about Buddha. Buddha was not very popular when he was alive but about 200 years after he died some people found all his writing and there were well over a thousand perhaps 13,000 and these people memorized them and then they were lost or destroyed. Why would someone destroy the writings of Buddha? Because Buddha explained writing is the problem. This is why in Buddhist traditions they teach with verbal communication. Their schools are centered around verbal communication. This is a contradiction for many of these wise beings. They were suggesting written language and reading were the problems yet they had to write and allow others to read the writing to communicate the problem and this in turn gave the impression to the sane it was not written language and reading that was the tree of knowledge.

The deeper meaning is these wise beings were using the invention against the ones who invented it or the ones who encouraged it if you like a supernatural view. They were using it's own weapon against it. So the written language is the problem and when one wakes up they have to use the written language to tell ones who are under the influence of it that the written language is the problem.

The sane would call that hypocritical but the ones who are awake aren't really big on laws and morals since they never have won and never will win. Everything is on the table and all is fair in this war. Everything is fair in the war. That's the only rule in the war. I happen to have an aversion to money but that's my problem. That's my flaw. Perhaps I will have to overcompensate in some areas to make up for that infinite flaw. Once one wakes up one will is going to understand one thing very swiftly. The sane are going to set traps for you. You keep your head and remind yourself who you are dealing with. - 11:14:42 PM

Chaos doesn't happen for a reason.

9/17/2009 6:06:54 PM – The sequential based education is like a fire. Thousands of years ago someone found this fire and it looked good to the eyes and was pleasing and so the mental doubt or questioning if it was perhaps too good to be true was overlooked. So everyone since it was initially found or invented never questioned if perhaps it was not as good and perfect as it appeared.

No one questioned that maybe this sequential education perhaps had some down side to it. So here were are thousands perhaps six thousand years later and still the powers that be are not questioning that perhaps this invention has a downside. It is as if we are the biggest suckers in the universe. We are so mentally broken we cannot even question that this education could have any flaws at all. We have silenced the right brain so harshly we do not have any ambiguity or doubt at all which is a right brain trait. I do not detect one single human being on this planet that has any business being around children while pushing this sequential education on them. They if anything should be locked up for the safety of the species.

These beings who push this sequential education on children should not be allow around children until they at least show signs of brain function, not intelligence just brain function. I do not ever expect them to show signs of intelligence I just would like to see signs of brain function so perhaps they would get to a mental level of understanding so they would stop mentally raping innocent children. Just wait till I start telling you how I really feel.

I do not care if they tell you they are god. I do not care if they tell you everyone voted for them. I do not care if they have all the weapons in the universe. You have them call me and I will convince them to get back in the pit they came from. I speak with people and I explain this situation and I can tell they try to use their sequential logic and they always talk their self out of the remedy. They es mortuus mentally quod illa idiots quisnam servo effectus is ut populus operor non mereo mereor ut spiritus procul totus. The ones who condition these beings into this state of mind leave people in this state of mind and they walk away and never tell them the remedy so they are worse than murders and rapists and molesters.

Of course this is hell so in hell the rapists and murders of children never get punished. Hell is simply the absence of righteousness. This society mentally rapes people so harshly the people cannot even understand they have been mentally raped so they cannot get out of it. The people wander aimlessly and their perceived purpose is foolishness. I am telling you I woke up to the fact I got mentally raped and I am telling you if you do not apply the remedy which is mental suicide you are in fact better off dead. You go apply the remedy and wake yourself up or you go jump off a cliff into the sea with a stone tied around your neck.

Ik heb geen eens begonnen te schrijven, om te vechten, om zicht te hebben.

You are complicit i meabhrach raping leanaí beaga. Cad a cheapann tú go bhfuil mo thuairim tú? Cad a cheapann tú mé ag dul a dhéanamh leat?- 6:29:22 PM

7:25:04 PM – When I wake up from sleep the heightened awareness is very strong. After I have been up for twenty hours or so I start to mellow out or the heightened awareness starts to diminish so I become rather docile and compassionate or I look at the situation with less urgency.

It is important to step back and look at this situation from a distance because at times one can get caught up in the hype. It does not make sense to me that other people could be this ignorant about this education. That does not pan out at times so I have to consider the other possibility. There can only be one actual reason I cannot communicate with other people properly. There can only be one true reason why it seems like everyone is asleep and I am awake. There can only be one possible reason why all of the sudden in the last ten months or so since the accident everything makes perfect sense to me. There can only be one possible reason why I am trying to make the entire world listen to me. There can only be one possible reason that I am trying to save the world from itself. That one possible reason is I am in fact dead and I am trying to come back to life but I cannot because I am dead.

I am in fact dead but I am physically alive. My mind has passed on and I have a strong craving to want to come back to the living but I cannot so I am trying to bring the living here to where I am at. That is really what is happening. It is not possible I could do some fear conditioning and reach a level of intelligence just from that. That does not make any sense. It is not possible a one second of fear conditioning, a near death experience could open up my mind to such a degree I am unable to find any difficulty understanding any comment any human being has ever said in all of recorded history. Is right brain that powerful once unveiled?

It is simply impossible that a near death experience or an altering of perception could create these kinds of results but it is possible that I mentally died and passed on and I am looking at the world from the other world and it all makes sense because hindsight is 20/20.

It is not even important if any of the living believe that because I am trapped here anyway. I have already died so this would explain why I am so detached from life itself. This would explain why I have no goals and have no cravings and have no ability to feel satisfaction or dissatisfaction. If I was alive I certainly would be taking advantage of all my new found intelligence and cashing in on it but I have no desire to do that. I would be trying to set myself up for a comfortable existence. I would be thinking about my future but I am not thinking about my future because I am not use to the fact my future is infinity.

I certainly would like to think because I am aware of this it would change something but the very nature of infinity is nothing does change. I am mocking the world because I am no longer in the world mentally. I cannot seem to find anyone I can relate to because everyone I know is still alive. I keep trying to say they are dumb because I cannot face the fact I am dead. I am trying to suggest they defeat their fear of death so they will die and so I will have company but that is not possible because one is alone in infinity.

I am trying to have company but I cannot have company so I am writing in hopes I can change that reality but I cannot change that reality. I killed myself and I am trying to blame it on others. I am bitter and angry and mean because I killed myself and I cannot take it back. I try to make it seem like the world made me kill myself but I made me kill myself. The world didn't kill me the world just does what the world has always done. I try to write these things down with the assumption I can now move on and I have closure but I cannot move on and their cannot be closure because the deed is already done.

A spirit is in infinity so it's logical it wants company. A spirit wants company but it cannot have company it can only have sensations of passing company. I should be afraid of things and I should be afraid to publish these books and I should be afraid to publish these books unedited and I should be afraid to tell people what I tell them but my mind will not allow me to be afraid.

My mind simply forgets what I have written and so I just keep writing and never can remember what exactly I write so I feel like I never have said enough. I try to reach the end of the writing and then I cannot remember what I wrote so I start all over again. I want to believe I am just having a moment of doubt but the truth is I have no moments of doubt just lots of moments of denial. I don't think this fear not conditioning has anything to do with psychology it in fact has to do with dying to yourself.

I know what the living are thinking because I was once alive but the living can never figure out what I am thinking because the living have not experienced death yet. I have to write infinite books no matter how much I try to talk myself out of it but no matter I say all I really understand is that I am dead. I am not alive because a live person has goals in the world and looks forward to the world and to having kids and having a love and having wealth. I have none of that. I am indifferent to the world. I am not of the world. I understand I can cause lots of mischief in the world with my words but that is not going to solve anything for me. The harsh words are simply a symptom I am not use to eternity yet. I am trying to come back to life by emulating ones who are alive. That is a logical approach to the problem. - 8:00:22 PM

8:08:37 PM – So perhaps there is a supreme being and he is in eternity and he finds us and starts to suggest ways we can join him in eternity because he wants company. So that is all this is about. Some entity that just wants company but can never really be satisfied or dissatisfied. So the entity tells us if you apply this fear not remedy and defeat your fear of death you will mentally die and come to eternity and be with him but once one is there they cannot detect the entity because one is in eternity also. This line would then negate existence all together.

There would be no point to existence at all if one simply mentally dies and leaves existence mentally or spiritually. This means religion is simply a cult of the living dead. Humans beings apply these techniques to in fact trick their self into dying before they die. So there are not any human beings who are really stupid or asleep there simply are no human beings who can ever be as wise as a being that is dead or in infinity. The living can never be as wise as the dead because the dead have the perspective of life and death. Perhaps I am relevant just not on this plane of existence called life. I can jump back on the fence much faster than you.- 8:22:16 PM

8:43:21 PM – So there are three spatial dimensions. X,Y and Z coordinates. Then there is the fourth dimension which is a temporal dimension which is time. Then there is a fifth dimension which is also a temporal dimension but the absence of time. It is similar to the time dimension because it is not measurable and it also is not absolute. So temporal means mental, or a cerebral dimension which means it cannot be traveled to by physical means only by cerebral or mental means. So the dimension after the first three cannot be travel to except mentally. So one can travel through time but not in a physical way only a mental way. In this fifth dimension there is no time so one is all time. There is no reason to go anywhere in a physical way because one can go anywhere on the mental 5th dimension.

Einstein explained a ship would need a gas tank the size of the universe to go the speed of light. This was explaining the speed of light can never be attained in the first four dimensions. In the fifth dimension which is a mental or cerebral dimension all the rules change. In the no time 5th dimension one can easily travel far beyond the speed of light because it is on a cerebral level. To ones in the first 4 dimensions this does not seem possible because their reality is based on the four dimensions. This is just like if there is a line in the first dimension it cannot relate to a line in the third dimension. A line in the first dimension will see a line in the third dimension as simply a flat line with no height or width. So a person in the fourth dimension is only able to relate to things on a physical level but in the fifth no time dimension the physical level becomes obsolete.

In the fifth dimension things that are impossible in the fourth dimension are effortless. Ones in the fourth dimension cannot see any value to being in the fifth dimension because they are looking for results on a physical scale which is what the three dimensions are based on. This works both ways because in the fifth dimension physical aspects are no longer important only cerebral aspects are important. So to travel back in time in using the fourth dimension it is impossible but in the 5th dimension it is only a matter of a thought so it requires no physical forces or aspects to achieve. The four dimensions bottle neck is the physical. The physical dimensions have an absolute limit but then in the fifth dimension there are no limits because everything is done on a cerebral none physical level.

A person in the fourth dimension needs to go to a destination so they buy a plane ticket and pack their luggage and make plans and travel this long distance to reach their vacation spot. A person in the fifth dimension simply thinks about that location and they are there. This cannot be comprehended by ones in the fourth dimension because their mind is under the influence of the forth temporal dimension which is time. In the fifth temporal dimensions no time, all the physical aspects disappear and there is only one form of travel and that is cerebral or mental travel so all of the barriers in the first fourth dimensions are removed. So going from the fourth dimension to the fifth dimension all the rules change so the rules no longer carry over to the fifth dimension so one actually transcends the limits caused by the spatial dimensions.

One in the fourth dimension has to physically go somewhere to feel like they have traveled and one in the fifth dimension does not even have to move physically to feel like they have traveled.

This creates a situation where the ones in the fourth dimension cannot grasp that and in the same manor ones in the fifth dimension cannot grasp why a person needs to travel physically to go to a destination. The rule is, something in a lower dimension cannot understand what a higher dimension is like but the higher dimension can understand what the lower dimension is like. So the dimensions are backwards compatible but not forwards compatible. - 9:31:34 PM

10:07:39 PM – So, this written education has mentally altered us and brought us from this fifth dimension to the fourth dimension. The early wise ones were simply trying to tell us this tree of knowledge did that to us and were trying to explain to us how to get back to this fifth dimension.

The whole reason modern day hunters and gatherer tribes care little about all the things society cares about is because they are in the fifth dimension. So death itself is the fifth dimension/eternity/ no sense of time and in order to reach that state of mind one has to defeat their fear of death or defeat death. This means perhaps god is death or god is no sense of time or god is the 5th dimension. The lords are the ones who can bring one closer to god. The lord tried to bring man back to god because man feel out of gods graces with this invention written language and went backwards to the 4th dimension from the fifth dimension and thus became very physically orientated and lost the cerebral orientation that is the 5th dimension. So when a person says I made peace with god when they are near death they mean they made peace with their own death or they let go of life so they go back to the fifth dimension just before they literally die.. - 10:17:44 PM

Now that I have thoroughly ruined this book I will try to gracefully finish it so I can start the 11th book. No wonder I give away my books because they all suck. When your books suck you pretty much have to be charitable.

10:23:52 PM – I draw in your sand, you can't understand. - 10:24:08 PM

Hanya satu dapat terjaga pada satu waktu. Aku tidak bisa tidur. Aku tidak bisa menangis.

10:58:44 PM – So people are in this left brain state and it makes them see everything as parts. So then there are cars and everyone

133

wants a different car so there are many kinds of cars and no one wants the exact same car.

Then there are many kinds of cars and so there are also many kinds of problems each car can have. There is no uniformity to the car design so there are many kinds of problems that go wrong and so there are many kinds of car accidents and thus there are many people who die because the cars are not uniform. If everyone saw things as one thing they would not be concerned if their car looked like everyone else's and so there would only be one kind of car and this car could be evolved to an extreme state of safety. It would look something like a bumper car. It would look horrible to the ones who only see parts and judge everything but it would be very safe.

The ones who only see parts keep insisting on these unsafe different cars and so they keep dying in these unsafe different cars and that is nature's way of taking care of keeping the population down. Nature deals with this mentally unsound species and makes them think things that eventually leads to them dying avoidable deaths.

The sane could easily have a very safe car and one that was nearly free of needing to be repaired but they would not be able to tolerate the fact it would look bad if they had the same car as everyone else and they think they are unique or special because they have a different car but in reality nature is making them make these poor choices so nature can get rid of them. There is no logical reason to drive eighty miles an hour but the sane perceive that is fun but in reality that is nature tricking them into situations where there is a good chance they will die. There is no logical reason to drive a motorcycle but the sane perceive it is fun but in reality it is nature tricking them into unsafe situations so they die. There is no reason to fight over dirt but that is nature's way of tricking the sane to kill their self off. There is no reason to take drugs to feel good because one of sound mind should feel good so that is nature's way of tricking them to kill their self off. There is no reason to kill each other over money but nature tells their unsound mind if they have money they will be happy so they kill each other off for money and they never end up happy, they just figure out another thing to make their self feel happy and have fun and eventually they die in that pursuit. This is what nature does to unsound creatures because nature does not like unsound creatures so it has a harmony and if that harmony is not met, trickery into death begins for that creature. There is no reason to kill the ecological system unless ones goal is to kill their self off and that is the goal. Of course the sane are not aware of this and they just chalk it up to unforeseen events but the events are not unforeseen they are obvious.

The events are simply many ways nature is tricking them to kill their self off because they are mutations that are not viable and thus are doomed to extinction. Nature cannot afford disharmony. It is similar to a checksum in a program file. The checksum is a long digit and when the program file is made this checksum is created and if that checksum is ever altered it means the program itself is compromised and therefore nonviable or altered from its original state and so it is suspicious or a potential threat so it must be replaced. - 11:16:22 PM

[Genesis 3:16 Unto the woman he said, I will greatly multiply thy sorrow and thy conception; in sorrow thou shalt bring forth children; and thy desire shall be to thy husband, and he shall rule over thee.]

So the sane have this unsound mind and so many things like pain are turned up to a great degree so the women suffer in child birth. The native tribes have children also but they can tolerate the child birth and they do not need drugs and they do not complain. Now the sane will go on and suggest "These tribes sometimes lose babies in child birth" and that is the whole point.

The sane try to save everything and have a god complex so they end up with nursing homes filled with people who lost brain function years ago and they still keep them alive as if they were alive. The sane try to defeat nature itself. The sane cannot accept nature and that is why nature cannot accept the sane. People are supposed to die or the population gets so great everyone dies. The sane hate that reality so they fight it and the more they fight it the more certain everyone is going to die from over population.

It is like a boat on the ocean and there is only enough room in that boat for a certain amount of people and so someone has to go out of the boat or the whole boat will sink. The sane hate that reality and none of them are willing to accept it because the sane hate nature. Nature knows best and when a human tries to create an artificial nature, nature does not play that game. What is happening in society outside of the mental rape of people by education is there are all the diseases and mental problem arising because there are simply far too many people and the more problems that arise the more complicated it gets until there is total meltdown. There will be total anarchy and it will be every man for himself and nobody's life will be valuable.

This is also a symptom of nature taking care of business. Society is under the influence of nature and not in control of nature so society is blind to the ways of nature. The sane will never opt out of having a child because they perceive it means they are of value. A child is a bench mark of success in society. The sane are so mentally unsound they will keep having children even when their own experts say "We cannot stand an increase in world population." The sane can never grasp what that even means because their mind is so out of whack they have a god complex and think they are above nature itself even though they are a product of nature. The sane are running towards the cliff and assume they will certainly survive the fall because of some miracle at the last second. The sane assume they can defy the laws of nature and that proves they are insane. - 11:39:46 PM

[Genesis 3:16 Unto the woman he said, I will greatly multiply thy sorrow and thy conception; in sorrow thou shalt bring forth children; and thy desire shall be to thy husband, and he shall rule over thee.]

This comment is beyond the sane one's ability to grasp because they take everything on face value. Their right brain pondering aspect is gone. This is not speaking about females this is saying after the education a person is a woman in relation to the serpent. They will be in great mental sorrow and have many desires. They simply will be mentally cursed. Perhaps neurosis would be a more accurate term. Perhaps hallucinating beyond understanding would be a more accurate term. Perhaps insane to the point they should be caged for their own safety and the safety of the children would be perfectly accurate. Adam was quite harsh in his comments. Perhaps he should be scolded. - 11:51:57 PM

136

9/18/2009 1:16:02 AM – What these ancient texts really are saying is a constant reminder of what we are. They are a reminder that keeps playing over and over in the mind. They have been playing over and over for thousands of years in our mind. These texts are tormenting us and mocking us and spitting on us and reminding us. They are like a tattoo on our foreheads that can never be taken away. Every time we look in the mirror we see that tattoo on our foreheads. We see the mark of the beast. I am in the same sinking boat you are in except I was not as hesitant to put my head under the water. I have pondered this one comment in these texts and I cannot deny it. I cannot escape it. I cannot stop it. You would be infinitely wise to not even read any further. I recall I suggested in earlier volumes one should not invade my personal diaries. I recall you were warned.

[Genesis 3:14 And the LORD God said unto the serpent, Because thou hast done this, thou art cursed above all cattle, and above every beast of the field; upon thy belly shalt thou go, and dust shalt thou eat all the days of thy life:]

[Genesis 3:15 And I will put enmity between thee and the woman, and between thy seed and her seed; it shall bruise thy head, and thou shalt bruise his heel.]

When one gets the education they are in fact the serpent and there is no remedy for the serpent, there are just varying degrees of hell. One can not apply the fear not technique and remain in the darkest depths of hell or one can repent and apply the fear not remedy and move on up to the 2nd or third level of hell but no matter what, one is in hell and one is the serpent. Upon thy belly thou shall go all the days of thy life. Only a serpent goes on its belly. So these texts are mocking the serpent and the serpent is anyone who got the education. So the education itself is the covenant with the devil. So the adults already got the education and so they are the devil and they get the children and educate them with the devils covenant and they make the children the devil also. So society is a satanic cult that takes innocent children and makes them the devil like the adults are the devil. So society itself is of the devil itself.

There is a story about the first time the Cherokee Indians tried to invent a language a written language and this was around 1820. The man who was working on this language had the symbols written on the wall and his wife came in and saw the symbols and said something along the lines of "That is the work of the devil." So the point is, this education itself is not of wisdom it is a way to make people the devil. The whole society and civilization is of the devil and the only ones who are not of the devil are the tribes who did not get the education and the devil is killing those tribes off. The devil looks at those tribes and tries to make them of itself and if they resist they are destroyed and that is the nature of the devil.

[Genesis 3:15 And I will put enmity between thee and the woman, and between thy seed and her seed; it shall bruise thy head, and thou shalt bruise his heel.]

Enmity means hatred and hostility. Males are hostile to women. The serpent is hostile to women. The males are the ones who got the education first. There will be hostility between the seeds which means the males will mate and create more potential devils with the woman. Bruised thy head means they will have the mark which means they will be mentally tainted. Bruise his heel means they will be in sorrow or it will be difficult for them to function as in walk mentally/think because their walking is hindered from the bruise.

[Genesis 3:24 So he drove out the man; and he placed at the east of the garden of Eden Cherubims, and a flaming sword which turned every way, to keep the way of the tree of life.]

And so God cast mankind out and so mankind became of the devil and this is because mankind embraced the tree of knowledge or the covenant with the devil and so the flaming sword to keep the way of the tree of life which means it kept man from going to the tree of life. And placed man at the east of the garden means that is the dawn or the cardinal point of when mankind fell from grace and embraced the devil.

Granted this is a supernatural take on the texts but the reality is the same. One cannot break the curse once they get the education, one can only reduce its bad side effects. One cannot go back to how they were before they got the education mentally. One can only try to reduce the suffering caused by it. There is no salvation there is only varying degrees of neurosis after one gets the education. I am pleased with the filler that made. I will go as deep as you want to go. Non podo crer que as persoas tratan a xente realmente espertar a esta realidade que debe ser totalmente tolo e sen corazón.- 1:56:24 AM

10:12:32 AM – Humans can adapt to any situation and that is perhaps our only redeeming quality. First thing about this situation we are in is population. We have nearly seven billion now so that's the first thing that we have to adapt to. This means stop having children. The problem is not we do not have enough people the problem is we have to get our minds out of this neurosis.

We start getting some people out of this neurosis and we will start having some good inventions, that's what is important not having more people to pity in neurosis. So the population is the bottom line start to this situation. If one cares at all about the species stop having kids. If one does not care at all about the species keep having kids but never complain about anything ever because you are a fool to begin with and get what you deserve.

The next step is to not educate some kids with this current education technique. Start educating some kids with just verbal education. This will allow some studies to give a contrast to how a person is when educated with the old methods and this new method. It's an experiment. Perhaps there are some parents who would sign up for this new method of education because they do not want their child mentally raped. Perhaps there are a couple of parents left on the planet who want their child to have brain function.

That's the whole plan. If those two aspects are not addressed it's all pointless. I am not negative I simply understand the solution is beyond the realms of the sane to ever apply. Simply put I know who I am dealing with. I am not dealing with people with a full deck. The sane are in some alien world of hallucinations and sequential logic. The problem is not as important as ones willingness to apply the solution.

So it's a two step process. Reduce the population and also start negating the neurosis. The right brain is very smart when unveiled so it will figure things out without any effort. That's the one thing we have on our side that is going to help us. The right brain has the creativity and the imagination and the random access thoughts and the ability to look at problems and come up with solutions at light speed. That aspect of the mind is the real solution here but if we keep locking it up in the next generation and this generation we are doomed. It is as simple as that. We are going to die off as a species if we do not get this right brain aspect back in the ball game. There is no greater truth than that. There is nothing in the universe more absolutely real than that fact. The education when not applied properly by people who have brain function does more damage to the mind than any other thing in known existence.

Drugs do great things for the mind in contrast to what the education does to the mind. Until one understands that reality they have no chance. I will just keep writing infinite books telling you the education ruins the mind if it is not applied properly until all you can think your mind is that. I will brainwash you back into consciousness just as you were brain washed into unconsciousness. No one is going to stop me because they do not have the mental function to stop me. And to some of these cults that suggest have lots of kids at all costs and never use birth control you shut your cursed mouth and I will remind you when you are allowed to speak, you aren't relevant anymore anyway. Your fruits are quite clear to me.- 10:35:05 AM

When all else fails, fail. The real point of all of this is we have six billion brilliant minds. Edison, Tesla, Einstein level minds right now we just have to wake them up. We just have to undo the damage this education has done to their mind and then everything else will sort itself out. There is no point in having more children since we have all the brain power we need right now we just need to get it functioning properly again since it has been turned off.

We have to turn on the light switch not have more kids. Having more kids so we can do to them what was done to us is meaningless and vain. Everyone is a brilliant genius they just have to apply the remedy and that takes one second. It takes one second to remedy this neurosis and it does not cost money and it does not take pills. It is a simple fix and a permanent fix. It takes no physical effort at all it is simply a one second mental decision at the proper time. Perhaps the sane cannot imagine it that simple because they like to make mountains out of flat ground. Whatever you have to tell yourself to apply the remedy you tell yourself. It does not matter what you have to tell yourself to apply the remedy just apply the remedy. - 11:00:23 AM

11:29:15 AM – I go to great lengths to avoid the inevitable war. I am in the appeasement phase. EGO sum trying ut causa per obscurum tamen EGO sum iam copiose conscius unus cannot causa per obscurum. Tunc is mos peto phase duos quod est accersitus Rutilus Mare. Perhaps some know what that means and perhaps some wish they didn't know what that means. I am actually neutral about that eventuality. - 11:34:35 AM

10:05:15 PM – A universitas vacuus vos taskmaster.- 10:05:51 PM

10:43:07 PM - I will now switch gears to anatomy to in hopes no one notices the 50k words I wrote before this part.

Thalamus - decides where to send incoming sensory data (from eyes, ears, mouth, skin)
 This is the processor of the sensory perceptions. It from a Greek word that means the room or chamber. That means everything one experiences comes here and this brain parts determines where to send it. This is a lot like a CPU in a computer. It gets data and determines what to do with it.

Sensory cortex - interprets sensory data
 This is a group or cortex. They have a lot to do with processing sensory information and then telling the brain what these senses or sensations mean. These cortex could be looked at like lenses and if there is dirt on the lenses then the information is going to be tainted. This is not on a physiological scale this is on a thought scale so any damage is intangible. The only way to determine damage is by ones

fruits or deeds or simply by how one act's. One example would be a person hears a song and they get very irritable and they say "I hate that music or that sound." That is an indication these sensory cortex are tainted. They are giving off the wrong impressions. A person should not be upset about a sound so these cortex are not working properly. This is carried over to words and sights and tastes.

The cerebral cortex is a mirrored structure. That means half is on the right hemisphere and half is on the left hemisphere. If one is conditioned to use the left brain with this education which is sequential based on just about every level it is just like a muscle. The left brain gets all the exercise and the right brain starts to become silent. After many years of the sequential education the right brain is very silent or veiled and the left brain is very strong and so this cerebral cortex mirror structure is very strong on the left and very weak on the right and this creates unbalanced lenses. This mirror structure should be equal but one side is very strong and one side is very weak in its function so the whole structure is unbalanced. This again is not physiological this is on a thought level.

This imbalance can only be determined by ones fruits or deeds or simply actions. If one has a strong sense of hunger and actually gets weak when they don't eat even after 12 hours their sensory cortex structures are out of whack. If one hates certain kinds of sound to the point it actually makes them mad their sensory cortex structures are out of whack. If one hates certain words which are also sounds it's because their sensory cortex structures are out of whack. Simply put their judgment is out of whack because their sensory cortex structures are unbalanced because they got all these years of left brain conditioning and the right brain aspect is weak. One can lift weights with their left arm and never lift weights with their right arm and eventually the mirror image or synchronization of the two arms will be out of harmony. The only difference is this imbalance is on a thought level not a physiological level so it cannot be measured by a machine so it can only be measured by the symptoms of actions one exhibits. Medicine cannot cure your thoughts it can only sedate you to the point of silencing those thoughts. Any way one wants to cut it, if a person gets many years of sequential left brain conditioning which is what education is, and they do not get an equal amount of right brain random access conditioning their mind itself can only be one thing, way out of balance.

Hippocampus - stores and retrieves conscious memories; processes sets of stimuli to establish context.

This part is associated with theta waves on an EEG and Theta waves are relative to when one is wide awake and also when one is dreaming. One who has been conditioned to the left may perceive being wide awake but not on an absolute scale of wide awake. Wide awake to a person who has applied the remedy and is in this 5th dimension in contrast to one who has not would be like a person who has not being on about 10 cups of coffee. Someone on the left is only wide awake relative to others on the left but they are in fact slothful relative to ones who have applied the remedy. The Hippocampus is also relative to certain psychological conditions such as memory loss and also Schizophrenia. It is difficult to detect Schizophrenia using physiological tests because the condition is really paranoia and hallucinations. Those symptoms are relative to the stability or harmony in the sensory cortex structures. If a person is sitting in the dark and they sense a ghost is coming to kill them and they run and turn on the light they are hallucinating and they are paranoid. Their cerebral cortex is playing tricks on them and they are believing it is reality and so they are a Paranoid Schizophrenic. This is the same with words. If a person believes saying a word will bring harm to them on a supernatural level they are paranoid and hallucinating.

If person believes if they look at a picture of nudity or a picture of a dead body they will be punished or be evil they are paranoid and hallucinating. Simply put a paranoid schizophrenic is a person who's mind is telling them things that are not true but that person believes it is true. A picture, the dark, or a word is not going to bring harm to you but if you think it will you are hallucinating because your sensory and thus cerebral cortex is not functioning properly and since it is on a thought level the only remedy is a thought conditioning remedy.

The left brain education is not a physical thing it is a thought conditioning and so the only remedy is a thought conditioning that counters all that left brain thought conditioning. Most of psychology is based on trying to solve a thought problem with a physical medicine and all that really does is postpone the symptoms but will never cure the symptoms. These psychological symptoms are not caused by the brain physiologically being damaged it is caused by the thought conditioning to the left to such an extreme and for such a long period the thoughts are imbalanced. If one works out the left brain and does work the right brain one is going to be very left brain heavy and education is all left brain, all of it. Every single class in the entire education system is sequential based left brain focused. It is impossible to go through all those years of sequential based left brain conditioning and come out with a sound mind. Aliens from mars will land long before the current education system produces one sound minded person from high school after all those years of left brain conditioning. That's the only reality you ever need to understand.

Perhaps you are starting to get the impression school makes people dumber not smarter and also makes them prone to fear and thus fear tactics. I would be pleased if that thought crossed your mind. A slave owner wants his slaves to be very scared because if not they may throw a rebellion or worse, escape. One can easily understand a world where most are afraid because that is this world it is a bit more difficult to understand a world where few are afraid.

A dog or cat will walk through a cemetery way out in the middle of nowhere at night and never even give it a second thought and it is not because they are stupid, it because they are not hallucinating because they did not get twelve years of left brain conditioning. Wild animals are not afraid of the dark because they are not hallucinating. I am pleased no one can understand anything I say ever. - 11:33:41 PM

4:16:17 AM – I am aware this letting go or fear conditioning is going to be the most important and difficult thing you ever do in your life. I am aware you did not put yourself in this situation. These aspects of the brain I am discussing are giving you false signals because you were conditioned way too far to the left as a child. The fear conditioning is the remedy and it is a onetime thing. There are many ways to half way do it but that's not good enough. There are ones who spend their whole life trying to reach this sound state of mind and they never do. This is why it is important to go the full measure. You do not want to get stuck half way. The full measure is facing perceived death and then making peace with it or allowing it. That is what those who lose their life will preserve it means. You are not going into an unsound state of mind you are going to a sound state of mind. Helen Keller explained it quite well.

'Death is no more than passing from one room into another. But there's a difference for me, you know. Because in that other room I shall be able to see.'

Helen Keller

Once you face your death and make peace with it by allowing it mindfully, not literally, you will in a few months go to another room and you will gain sight. That left brain state of mind you are in is going to try to talk you out of it. That left brain is going to say it's not safe because all these brain aspects I am talking about are giving you false signals. They are not working properly because you were conditioned into left brain to such an extreme you cannot even think clearly.

All of the things going on in your mind are not supposed to be going on in your mind. Whoever educated you did not know what they were doing and whoever educated them did not know what they were doing. There are no fear conditioning classes and there are no right brain counter conditioning classes to counter the left brain sequential conditioning classes. There is no such thing in the school system so that is why you are in this spot now and I am not suggesting it is your fault.

It is some one's fault but that is not important right now. I have plans for them. A lot of the things you read in these poorly disguised diaries you are simply not going to fully understand. There are also things going on in these diaries I do not fully understand. That is not important right now either. Once you get that fear out that right brain is going to power up and it will do the work for you. You will not have to do anything after this fear conditioning event. Whatever your mind is telling that is more important than this waking up is simply not true. I would not tell you that if it were not true. I am not concerned about what the experts say about what I say. They all had their chance and they were not up to snuff. They are the mentally blind leading others to be mentally blind. I am not suggesting there are a thousand in neurosis I am suggesting there are six billion in neurosis.

The mental arguments you are going to have against doing this are only going to be sequential elementary deductions and they are all going to fall short and be false. This conditioning is mental but you are going to have to believe it is physical death you are facing. That remedy is a symptom of what the adults did to you as a child. That remedy is a symptom of what the adults did to those adults when they were children. None of them knew what they were doing. That is not important, I have plans for them. Letting go means you join the team that may never win.

I don't see that we can ever win against them. That's what humility is, joining a team you know ahead of time has never won. They count on me but I can't do it. They say things to me and I cannot tell them I unable to win for them. No one has ever won. It's all just a string of attempts. Look what the sane do to the children. Look what the sane did to us. I will keep writing until I drop and the sane will mock that because they do not have the eyes to understand what that means. - 5:06:18 AM

"Because in that other room I shall be able to see.'

7:42:56 AM – [Exodus 32:19 - And it came to pass, as soon as he came nigh unto the camp, that he saw the calf, and the dancing: and Moses' anger waxed hot, and he cast the tables out of his hands, and brake them beneath the mount.]

This is the problem. Once a person is conditioned they cannot tell they are in neurosis. Moses brought all these people out of the cities but many of them got the education conditioning and did not apply the remedy. That was his fatal mistake. He saw the calf means he saw people who were still under the influence of the conditioning or neurosis and "dancing" is a symptom and "calf" is a symptom of behavior. So Moses freed the people but brought in a bunch of the sane with them and so he tainted the pool so to speak. So his anger waxed hot because he knew he blew it. Throwing the rules/tablets away shows he could not win or all bets are off or anything goes.

This is the history between Abraham and Mohammed. Abraham told people the fear not remedy and they understood it and things were looking up for a while then Moses came along later and things were getting out of control again. People stopped applying the remedy and still used the written language. Then all the people from the time of Moses to the time of Jesus stopped applying the remedy and so things were way out of control again. Then after Jesus people forgot again to apply the remedy and then Mohammed came along and things were impossibly out of control. This is a symptom of how subtle this sequential education is to the mind.

Subtle is an important aspect to this. The people who get the education and the people who get the education and apply the remedy look exactly the same but their deeds or fruits are different which are thoughts and actions. This comment sums up this subtle aspect.

[Genesis 3:1 Now the serpent was more subtil than any beast of the field which the LORD God had made. And he said unto the woman, Yea, hath God said, Ye shall not eat of every tree of the garden?]

This comment is saying "What is wrong with written language it looks good to me?" and then the response is "Yes, how can anything be wrong with the pretty language that makes one wise?" The conditioning achieved in learning this invention is very crafty but its impact on the mind is very harsh. I will throw every single argument in the universe at the sane and the vast majority will still not believe they have been conditioned mentally into an unsound state of mind. And then it goes deeper.

Eventually even if everyone understands that, society will forget that and stop applying the remedy and the next generation will forget the remedy all together. This is a symptom of how subtle the conditioning is. This is how history works. Once in a blue moon a person wakes up and they are deemed to be a genius or wise man but what really is happening is once in a blue moon someone wakes up from the neurosis and they stick out. They are not wise men they are of sound mind and the sane cannot imagine that because if they are of sound mind then that means the entire society is insane. One can just simply think back on history at every single creative genius there ever was and what they really see is a human being who broke out of the neurosis to one degree or another and reverted back to a point of sanity before they got the sequential education conditioning. That's a reality the sane will never understand.

The sane have the definitions of words all wrong. The words Prophet and Saint are simply people who woke up from the neurosis to a varying degree. The sane will deny that because that would mean they are mentally trashed and their ego which is encouraged by the left brain conditioning will never allow them to admit that to their self. It's not really important what the sane think because the sane are the sane. Everything they do is sane. The sane mentally rape defenseless children and then brag to everyone how well they educated them and also brag how much they care about children.

The sane will actually mentally condition children and then say they care about children. They are text book definition of insane. An insane person can kill people literally and not even be aware they did it. That's why they are called the sane because if anyone who is awake calls them by their real name they will freak out and kill them.

I am no such fish. I am the hunter and the gatherer and if the sane get in the way they get hunted and gathered. The sane call the ones who are awake crazy because if they didn't call them crazy it would mean they are crazy and they do not have the imagination of right brain to figure that one out. I am on this fence. I try very hard to keep the line that this written language just put us all in neurosis inadvertently but sometimes I learn the other way on the fence and I start to get the impression they are possessed by the devil incarnate. Some who are awake are certain which one of those two it is, I however am not yet at that level of intelligence. It is certainly one or the other or one in the same.- 8:26:49 AM

11:40:59 PM – This left brain state of mind the years of sequential conditioning creates makes one an addict and the drug is emotions. One simply becomes an addict to emotions and they exhibit the exact same symptoms a drug addict exhibits.

The emotions are turned up to such an extreme because of this left brain conditioning one becomes addicted to all the emotions.

Some people love to feel good and some people love to feel bad. Some people love the feeling of depression and some people go to great lengths to always feel good. The problem with that is one is just like a drug addict and they have to come down sometime. A person is simply on a roller coaster emotionally. That is what a drug addiction is, a roller coaster.

A person falls in love and feels great then the relationship ends and they feel like death. The love and depression afterwards are not even the point, it's the emotions that one seeks. Some love to be scared and some love to feel safe. Both of these are emotions and they are drugs. Some like to be accepted and some like to rebel, these are also emotions and also drugs. Some will say they are on top of the world and what they really mean is they are getting ready to fall.

Some say I feel great and what they mean is they are high on a drug called emotions and they are getting ready to fall. Some get in an argument and they get angry and those emotions are the drug. The problem with all addiction is a person starts acting in ways to encourage that addiction and not in logical ways. A person will treat another person unfairly in order to make a buck in order to feel good emotionally because they feel good when they have money. That is a symptom of a person doing something to feed their addiction to emotions.

A person addicted to these emotions as a child as a result of the education may never be able to kick that habit. They will suggest the emotions are needed just like a drug addict thinks the drug is not harming them. This denial is expected in any addiction. They have talked their self into believing these emotions are needed to survive just like a heroin addict talks their self in believing heroin is need for them to survive. These addicts will do anything to feel emotions. They will go hunting and kill animals to feel emotions. They will insult others to feel emotions. They will kill others to feel emotions. They will eat certain foods to feel emotions. They will do actual drugs to feel emotions. They will give gifts to feel emotions. They will do various things to be regarded by their peers in order to feel the emotions. The emotions type is not even important because very person who is addicted has certain emotions they crave. - 11:56:28 PM

9/20/2009 4:02:46 PM – Filler is important.

[Exodus 32:2 And Aaron said unto them, Break off the golden earrings, which are in the ears of your wives, of your sons, and of your daughters, and bring them unto me.

3 And all the people brake off the golden earrings which were in their ears, and brought them unto Aaron.

4 And he received them at their hand, and fashioned it with a graving tool, after he had made it a molten calf: and they said, These be thy gods, O Israel, which brought thee up out of the land of Egypt.]

One aspect of this comment is relative to what is known by the sane as the age of metal. Bronze age and the like. There is the stone age the bronze age and the iron age. The tribes in the Amazon are still in the stone age and this is not relative to intelligence this is relative to luxury. The actual metal ages came into being somewhere around 3000 to 5000 BC. This again is in direct relation to when written language was invented. From one perspective it appears that these metal working ages made us much smarter but in reality they made us rely on luxuries and in turn made us more dependent on luxuries and thus less reliant on our minds. If a hunter had to kill a deer for food with a stick they would have to be very clever in their methods and if a hunter just has to point a gun at that deer from 200 yards away they can pretty much be blind and they will still get lucky once in a while.

The deeper reality of this is destruction. If a person has to catch a fish with their hands it will take a while for them to catch all the fish but if they use a huge net they can wipe out the population of the fish swiftly. If a person goes to war against others and they have to throw stones at them it's possible no one would even die in that war but if they use an atomic bomb they can wipe out lots of people in a moment. This is also relative to being separated from the actual killing and then the killing seems like it's not even real.

In a current conflict if the warring factions had to fight with their hands there would not be very many people signing up to fight that war because it would be far to personal. Instead we have guns and bombs that can kill from great distances and so the killing is not very personal and thus one can kill far more people that way before losing their mind from doing so. This is all relative to these metal ages. It seems like these metal ages really helped us but in fact they made us rely on material things instead of our minds. One proof of this is what the sane call wilderness survival courses. To actually be in a mental state that one has to be taught how to survive in the wilderness when in fact they are a wild animal to begin with can only be described as vanity.

What this wilderness survival training is a symptom of is human beings are domesticated to the point they are no longer viable as a creature in the wild. The sane are in this state of mind that living in nature is some scary unwanted situation but in reality that is their natural habitat but they have been mentally altered to such a degree they can no longer survive in their natural habitat so they must be kept in their cages. This is exactly what happens to zoo animals. The zoo animal is raised in a cage so long they can no longer survive in their natural habitat so they are no longer what they are. They are no longer a monkey that can live in its natural habitat they are simply a creature that can only be taken care of. They become a burden even to their self.

The sane may attempt to use sequential elementary logic and suggest "So we should all go back to the wild." but the reality is, they cannot. They can no longer be a human being because human beings can easily survive in the wild and the sane cannot easily survive in the wild so they are not really human beings by the definition of a real human being. The mind of the sane has been so drastically altered by the education they are no longer viable as a species. This is why nature is their weakness. Nature use to be human beings home and now it is their worst nightmare.

"No human being will ever know the Truth, for even if they happen to say it by chance, they would not even known they had done so."

Xenophanes

Understanding truth requires one to be able to detect lies.
Truthful illusion and illusion of truth are not truth.
Truth is often a well disguised lie.

Cerebral truth and material truth never see eye to eye.
Settling on a truth only proves one has given up on finding truth.
It is far easier to be true to one's self than truthful to one's self.
When one can no longer question an answer they have found truth.
A mind is not always ready for the truth but the truth is always ready for the mind.
It is better to ask questions than mock answers.

'God is one, greatest of gods and men, not like mortals in body or thought.'

Xenophanes

Being in the experiment denotes one cannot understand the experimenter.
A scientist does not need to prove he is running an experiment.
An experiment is more important than the reasons for it.
The nature of God and the God of nature are indistinguishable.
You should be careful about one's who say they understand God because you might start believing you understand God also.
The truth about God is a truth we cannot understand.
When in an experiment it is best to understand what acting natural is.

"As the builders say, the larger stones do not lie well without the lesser."

Plato

The pebbles do not like the weight of a boulder.
Fearlessness often defeats the fearful.
A pebble is easily washed away in a shallow stream but a boulder can raise the level of the stream and keep the pebbles from washing away.
An unbalanced mind is a pebble that crumbles under pressure.

"And what, Socrates, is the food of the soul? Surely, I said, knowledge is the food of the soul."

Plato

Understanding often requires no teacher and knowledge often leads to misunderstandings.

Knowledge denotes memorization; Understanding denotes heightened awareness.

"Death is not the worst that can happen to men."

Plato

Being alive is more relative to thinking than breathing.

Mental death is the only escape from an unbalanced mind; Physical death is the only reward to an unbalanced mind.

An unsound mind is harder to live with than death.

With an unsound mind life is unsound so death is a bound.

An unsound mind is in a box long before it is buried.

"Wise men speak because they have something to say; Fools because they have to say something.'

Plato

Wise men are only detected by wise men but fools are detected by all.

It is difficult for a wise man to explain wisdom and more difficult for a fool to understand it.

Some think about thinking and some think they can think.

A wise man see's a loss as a chance for an understanding and a fool see's a loss as a chance to give up.

A wise man tries to make fools wise and fools try to stop him.

A wise man is simply a fool that has died and a great fool loves himself too much to become wise.

A fool see's a wise man as a fool and that is why a fool is not wise.

The wise see a fool as a candidate for wisdom but fools seldom understand that.

Fools cannot shield their self from wisdom but they often misunderstand it.

Minimus vereségek az Dyr.

"Comedy is very controlling - you are making people laugh."
Gilda Radner

A word is a grunt that can lead to war or peace but its best when it leads to more grunts.

Since the sane cannot live in nature they continue to destroy nature and replace it with this artificial nature called civilization. The sane will suggest life is much easier now with all these inventions but in reality what they are saying is "Now I do not even have to have a mind and I can survive."

The sane have traded their mind for their luxuries. This is why some people become very depressed and determine life is not worth living and they are correct. Life is not about luxury and so when there is so much luxury there is no life. The sane have determined as long as they can sit in their little cage and be fed and taken care of by all their metal inventions they are living life. The sane have determined as long as they keep growing in number they are living life when in reality the fact they keep growing in number proves they have no sense of sound harmony in their thoughts anymore. This is a symptom of the god complex they have in this extreme left brain state of mind. The sane actually believe they are more important than a tree or a bird or an earthworm but without those things there are no humans. The sane have lost sight of the fact they are a part of this machine called nature. The sane believe they are above the machine called nature and that is why nature has to correct their delusions.

Living a full life in a cage is not living. The native tribes who live in the Amazon have never spent the night in a house, have never been to the dentist, have never had an inoculation against disease, have never used soap to bathe and also have never had an operation to alter their facial features so they would like their self. This is an indication one of these two types of human beings, the tribes and civilized are very mentally unsound and not even in the realm of being viable as a living creature.

The actual left brain state of mind the written language has created in the sane is why they have all these problems, simply because their mind is no longer sound. One example is the Black death plague.

This plague was a direct symptom of the cities. This kind of plague was a symptom of the cities crowed conditions on one hand and in nature there are no crowded conditions. Then on a deeper level it effected beings who had an unsound mind and this unsound state of mind causes nervousness and stress and that means their immune system was compromised. One might suggest these tribes in the Amazon would not kill their self if they lost their job yet the sane do it on a daily basis.

The sane lose their mate and are mentally depressed for years and sometimes never recover. The sane will be in a relationship and their mate may leave them or scorn their love and then that initial mate may kill that one who left them. That is because they are in such extreme neurosis they can no longer even think clearly.

The sane have this scale of acceptability and if that scale falls out of balance it is time for them to lash out at either their self or at the ones they perceive caused their scale to swing out of balance. This is because they are no longer able to survive on their own. They are animals in cages and they simply cannot survive on their own merits. The sane are no longer a viable living creatures, they are simply a creature that has been conditioned to only being able to live in a cage.

If all of civilization disappeared these sane would simply die off because they could not survive on their own merits. Their minds could not take the shock of such a large change because left brain hates change. This means the sane like this tiny circle of comfort and if at any time this tiny circle of comfort is altered they panic. This panic is the result their genius right brain that loves to adapt to change has been veiled to such an extent the sane are simply unable to adapt to change. This creates situations where the sane see problems when there is no problem. The sane have been robbed of half of their mind and the complex, concentration, problem solving aspect of their mind and so they can no longer think their way out of simply problems and so they become frustrated and panic and come to very harsh conclusions. The sane are a slave to their conditioned unsound mind and they can ever escape that reality without a massive shock that allows their mind to break free of this left brain extreme cage they are trapped in. - 4:53:42 PM

5:04:43 PM –

[Exodus 32:8 They have turned aside quickly out of the way which I commanded them: they have made them a molten calf, and have worshipped it, and have sacrificed thereunto, and said, These be thy gods, O Israel, which have brought thee up out of the land of Egypt.

9 And the LORD said unto Moses, I have seen this people, and, behold, it is a stiffnecked people:]

So this word molten calf has many definitions. First off the written language is the calf the tree of knowledge. That what made human extreme left brained and hindered their mind or veiled their right brain so then they had to start making inventions to make up for that. That led to the metal ages. "Sacrificed and worshipped it" denotes the sane stopped using their minds and relied instead on these inventions. They sacrificed their own offspring to these inventions. The deeper meaning is, "What was wrong with us in the first place that we needed all of these things?" We lived for perhaps longer than 200,000 years without all these inventions and now we have to have them, people? If it was not broken why did we try to fix it? That is the absolute problem. We tried to fix something that was not broken and in turn ruined it. Leave well enough alone comes to mind.

The comment "stiffnecked people" is great humor. Stiffnecked is simply saying ignorant and ignorant is saying stupid and stupid is saying unsound mentally, stubborn. The sane are afraid of change because they no longer have the mental complexity to deal with uncertainty and change so they become bullheaded and thus stiffnecked. I guess the only advice I could ever give to the youth is;

No matter what do not try to be like your parents or the adults and make sure whatever they do, you do the reverse. The youth should look at the sane adults as a perfect example of what they never ever want to become. EGO mos moneo juvenis ut EGO deprehensio vel a tenuis testimonium of intelligence oriundus adults inter sanus. - 5:16:43 PM

6:02:42 PM – If every person does what is best for them then the group of people suffer. If every person does what is best for them and the group there is a certain harmony that is achieved. The problem with that is what a person thinks is best for them is not ever going to be what is best for the entire group because everything is relative to the observer. The means harmony itself is not about everyone winning. Harmony is about creating situation where loss and gain are equal or in harmony.

When a person is conditioned in this extreme left brain state they perceive loss is bad and with too many losses and they become depressed. When they become too depressed they do very drastic things and sometime kill their self and that in turn is what the harmony is all about.

If every creature always won then the harmony would be way out of balance and the ecological system would not function. The sane believe death is evil but in reality death is as valid as life. Losing is as valid as winning in a harmony system. The sane believe the longer a person lives the better but that is only relative to their belief living long is a symptom of winning.

On a larger scale, an ecological scale living as long as one can at all costs is devastating. One problem with this large brains humans have is that is has enabled them to actually negate the natural ecological balance in life. This appears like a good thing but it is a bad thing. When the ecological harmony is lost the entire harmony system breaks down and this means there is going to be some major consequences because harmony is always going to seek harmony. On a small scale a group of humans will assume that as long as they live long they are winning but then nature is going to throw some equalizer into the mix and many humans will die off because of it.

On this larger time scale then the humans did not really live longer they only ensure many will eventually live and die swiftly. A room with a million humans will not survive as long as a room with 2 humans in it. This is because a human conditioned too far to the left has this egotistical god complex side effect. The room with two people can work out some form of harmony much easier than a room with a million conflicting perspectives. A family has conflicts and then a neighborhood has conflicts, and then a city has conflicts, then a state and then the world. The greater amount of people involved the more likely conflicts will arise. This will eventually lead to groups who have like ideals fighting groups with contrary ideals.

One example is ones who are pro life fight with ones who are pro choice. The reality is neither group is pro life or pro choice they simply latch onto this ideal and find a contrary group and fight with it. This is relative to the god complex this left brain state of mind creates, simply put, seeing everything as parts. The pro life people hate harmony because they want life at any cost when in a harmony system, life and death must be kept in balance or the entire ecological system collapses and so in fact they are pro choice because they are ensuring the death of the species. They are unable to see very far because the left brain sequential logic is never able to go from beginning to end like the right brain random access can. They see a few steps and then make this conclusion and it is a half step conclusion.

This is all a symptom of how this education has altered our mental ability to think clearly. We tend to go to great lengths to fight for these ideals that are flawed to begin with but no one in the pro life group can understand what they are suggesting. They all believe a human life is more important than all other life but they are unable to fully understand without all other life human life is not sustainable. The ones who are pro choice are at least in the realm of reality because they are aware the population is way out of control, to a degree. Simply put we cannot sustain these numbers for very long. We cannot feed everyone as it is and at the same time people are still having more children. This again is the self centered god complex this left brain state of mind creates. As a species we need to start letting some people die not trying to save them. As a species we need to get off of this "save people at all costs" god complex. It is not panning out and it is going to be the doom of us.

By attempting to save everyone at any cost the sane are actually killing the species. The sane are not saving people they are killing everyone because there is way too many people as it is. China is aware of this. The whole world only sees parts so they sit around and think 'Oh that's just in China, we have manageable numbers in our country." China is in fact human beings and they understand there are too many humans and in fact are making humans by law stop reproducing and the whole world should be doing the exact same thing because they do not count the world population by countries they count the world population as one species and they understand it is getting way out of hand.

The sane have misunderstood some of the religious texts and they get the impression death is evil so they go out of their way to avoid it and in turn doom the entire species. There is one "race" of humans thinking they need a bigger population to protect them from another "race" of humans and so both groups keep overpopulating. This is because neither "race" understands they are the same species because they are conditioned into such extreme left brain they only see parts. This of course in not reversible until the whole species remedies this left brain state of mind caused by education, and since they species as a whole continues to condition the next generation into this extreme left brain state and never applies the remedy the entire species is doomed.

This is all a symptom that this education has turned us into a mentally unsound species and an unsound species is not viable and so we are in fact suicidal in nature. The species is suicidal in all of its actions but believes it is not suicidal in all of its actions and that is exactly what is suppose to happen because nature in its own way is going to take care of unviable creatures one way or another to restore harmony in the ecosystem. The species kills off all of the oceans and forests and other species and then goes around believing everything will work out, because some great supernatural being is going to come down and save them.

That is what nature wants the unsound species to believe. Nature wants the unsound species to feel a comfort zone because if that species felt they were in danger they would only last longer. So from the time of this left brain conditioning invention about 5400 to 7000 years ago we as a species have essentially been approaching a breaking point. On a scale of time that is a very short period for our species to go from harmony to extinction prone. This is an indication of how devastating this unsound state of mind is to our species. It is similar to a heroin addict who is near death from doing drugs for many years but when the heroin is offered they do not hesitate to take it again. Over 2500 years ago some wise beings simply said this tree of knowledge invention is going to kill you and here we are all this time later and we still have no clue what that means, and we even have complete systems of education set up now to indoctrinate the next generation with this mental destruction. This is all because this unsound state of mind has made us a suicidal species.

We kill ourselves every day and even the next generation and we do not have the mental faculties to understand that. That is the price of mental disharmony and that is the way nature takes care of mentally unsound and non viable species. This tree of knowledge invention was fatal to our species and even by saying that the species will mock that and laugh at that because they are in a suicidal state of mind and they are not even aware of it. If one does not believe this education is fatal all they have to do is contact someone in education and tell them you believe it conditions people into extreme left brain unsound state of mind and actually harms a person and you will be laughed off the face of the earth and told you are crazy.

This is the same response a person who is addicted to drugs will give you when you approach them about their addiction. The word is denial. Perhaps I am of unsound mind because I am not explaining this with greater urgency. Perhaps if I cared I would be explaining this to the sane using the only methods the sane understand, violence.- 6:50:13 PM

Society idolizes the great thinkers in history because they could do the one thing the sane can no longer do, think. Intelligence is not determined by the words one can spell properly, intelligence is determined by ones mental ability to question what everyone tells them is truth. If one cannot think for their self they certainly cannot think for others. One who is afraid of their thoughts is afraid of everything. One who is afraid of others thoughts is afraid of their own thoughts. Understanding one has misunderstood is definitive proof one may be thinking. Understanding one misunderstood offers rewards ignorance cannot provide. Thinking has more to do with observation than judgment. Quisnam can servo nos nobis. - 8:44:14 PM

I can't lose my battle and I can't win yours. Total blindness is clinically defined as NLP which is no light perception.

9/21/2009 3:01:21 AM –

There are some that never learn and unto them is the burn.

To the ones who understand the ones that build upon the sand.

The war is not over yet, so fight that you may not regret.

If you were a grain of sand I would offer my right hand.
-3:01:21 AM

5:39:11 PM – Applying the remedy may seem like this top of the mountain solution or the end of the road. Who doesn't want to have a sound mind and telepathy and feeling through vision and concentration abilities that can only described as unnamable? This makes it seem like the remedy is some great feat. Waking up as the result of applying the fear not remedy is a piece of cake. That is not what the battle is that is only you signing up for the team that never wins. Applying that remedy means you are signing up for the team that gets butchered for telling the truth, and that is being very optimistic.

One is going to have to have an argument in explaining this neurosis. One is going to have to understand psychology, neurology, anatomy, religion and have an argument relative to all of these topics. One is going to have to have an answer for every question the sane ask relative to this neurosis and that is not good enough. One is going to have to be flawless and that is not good enough. One is going to understand the definition of impossibility. One is going to understand being aware of what the sequential education does to one's mind and especially a child's mind does not mean anything to the sane. One is going to understand the definition of they know not what they do. One is going to wake up and understand who they are surrounded by. One is going to have to get use to getting their teeth kicked in mentally every single day and the days last a thousand years.

Once one is awake and aware of these things they are going to want to run and hide. One is going to try to find an escape hatch. One is going to find there are no escape hatches. There are two kinds of players on the team that never wins. There are those who talk their out of playing and those who can't wait to get mentally kicked in the teeth again.

This is why the remedy is nothing in contrast to the battle you are never going to win after you apply the remedy. The definition of humility is trying as hard as you can with the understanding you will never ever win on this team. It is not about having a good argument and it is not about saying the right things at the right time. When all is said and done the sane are going to ask "What is the remedy?" and that is when all your efforts fall apart.

Some people suggest meditation and that is a slow route and a safe route because suggesting "those who lose their life will preserve it." sounds very scary to the sane.

Suggesting submit to perceived death when you are in a situation you perceive death is also very scary to the sane. Of course the sane are afraid of bad haircuts so that is not a surprise. The sane are afraid of words and you are telling them to submit to their fear of perceived death. You are telling the sane to go pull an Abraham and Isaac and they do not like the sound of that.

In the East they try to suggest mediation but they do not exactly come right out and tell you what to mediate on. Being mindful of death is what the focus of the mediation is. In the west that would be a person who is suicidal. Meditation is really watching your thoughts and emotions mentally and then denying them or allowing them to pass mentally. So it is a form of detachment. Of course pulling and Abraham and Isaac or submitting to perceived death and lose your life to preserve it, is also a form of detachment. There is no greater form of detachment than to perceive you will die and then be meek and allow it, that is what letting go is and also what meek and humble is.

All of these strategies are saying the exact same thing and they are all attempts to wake up the sane from the neurosis caused by many years of sequential conditioning called the tree of knowledge. The point is, once one wakes up they will be obligated to explain this and they are going to understand the word vanity swiftly. One who is awake is not capable of being depressed or happy they will just be aware of this situation. One is going to try to deny this obligation and one will try to talk their self out of it. This battle of the minds is perhaps not cut out for everyone who wakes up. This is an indication of this suggestion going the full measure. One can certainly reach this state of mind and negate the remedy to an extent using mediation but the problem with that is one may not go the full measure. That is relative to this aspect of the brain.

Hypothalamus - activates "fight or flight" response
After the left brain conditioning this part of the brain is not functioning properly on a thought level. Physiologically it looks fine but it is not function properly. The Abraham and Isaac story is about Isaac not running, which is the flight aspect of fight or flight, when he saw that knife held over him. So Isaac submitted when this Hypothalamus was telling to run. Isaac chose to lose his life and thus preserved it. This is a mental technique to get this Hypothalamus working properly again. So in the East the strategy is to sit in a cemetery and mediate and this Hypothalamus is going to be sending lots of signals that tells a person to flee and they are not going to flee, and this silences this Hypothalamus and that means it starts function properly again and is not so hyperactive. This is what self control is.

This Hypothalamus is telling a person to run like the wind, a ghost is coming to kill you and then one applies self control and does not run and so they stop these false signals coming from this Hypothalamus and it starts working properly again. So all these years of left brain sequential conditioning has made this Hypothalamus start acting strange and that effects the entire mind. Of course that is a good thing for a taskmaster because he wants his slaves to be as afraid as possible so they will stay on the tread mill as it were. - 6:32:23 PM

11:10:14 PM – Some of this line of thinking is going to include patterns and right brain good at patterns. Carbon is atomic number 6 on the table of elements. It takes the carbon atom about 5700 years to decay. Written language was invented around 5400 to 7000 years ago. Carbon 12 isotope last forever. Carbon 12 isotope has 6 electrons, protons and neutrons. Human beings like all animals on the planet are carbon based. Carbon is an atom and an atom is mass and mass is physical or matter.

There is a comment about "in the flesh". The flesh denotes in this carbon based form. The tricky part is the written language conditions one into an unsound state of mind and they become very physically focused as in their physical appearance and having lots of physical wealth and what that means is the cerebral aspect of thoughts are diminished.

So this Demotic(written language) and math being very sequential based have conditioned us in this state of left brain where we are very aware of the carbon aspect of our being or of physical reality, so we are left looking around saying physical, matter is all that is real because we have turned down the cerebral aspect of our awareness inadvertently with this invention called demotic and math.

So we are in a universe that is very physical or it has atoms and atoms are mass. Then on this other level we have very powerful brains and when one is mentally sound they are very cerebral. This cerebral aspect suggests one is more focused on thoughts and thinking than on actual physical aspects because a person can only be one or the other, and cannot be both at the same time because as one increases the other decreases.

For example going to the moon is a physical desire and to one in a cerebral state it means nothing because it has nothing to do with the cerebral world. To one in the physical state of mind world, money means a lot because money is a means to buy physical things but to one in the cerebral world money does not register because it is physical.

Climbing a mountain is something one in a physical state of mind would desire and to one in the cerebral state of mind it would be meaningless. To one in the physical state of mind building a pyramid would be of value and perhaps even demonstrate power in the physical world but one in the cerebral world that pyramid would mean nothing. So to one in the physical state of mind building that pyramid would be of value and to one in the cerebral state of mind building that pyramid would be vanity. One in the physical world would value life or at least their own because without life they have no physical world to experience. On the contrary one in the cerebral mind set would not be afraid of death because to them loss of physical aspects would not mean anything because they are so cerebral they are not attached to the physical world anyway. So this conditioning into extreme left brain has made us very materialistic and in turn has silenced our cerebral aspects.

So in contrast to the tree of knowledge, we were in the cerebral state of mind so we hunted and gathered because we were not prone to materialism. We didn't need a house to attach to, we could just pick up and move at any moment and it did not bother us. Another way to look at it is in this cerebral state of mind before the education is we had no problem with change because we had the cerebral faculties to deal with change. So these tribes who did not get the education and were in a cerebral state of mind looked rather barbaric because they were not physically focused in relation to materialism simply because they were more focused on cerebral aspects. So the warning about the tree of knowledge was simply saying "If you embrace this written language and math you will go into a physical based state of mind and everything will change as a result."

So then there was Abraham who burned down the cities because the cities were indication we went from cerebral focus mentally to physical focus mentally or materialistic focus. Then after this, economics started kicking in, so to speak. Monetary systems started kicking in to buy all the physical products that everyone wanted all the sudden. The problem with this physical focused mindset is one can never have enough and as one tries to have enough they destroy the physical things around them that are required for them to remain viable. This would include the ecological system, forests and animal populations. The problem with that is once those are diminished to a great degree the human species dies and that is actually suicide.

If one cuts off the hand that provides their way to survive they in fact commit suicide. So the mark of the beast would be someone who is physically or materialistically orientated and this would be obvious because they are focused on material things(666 = matter, carbon 12 isotope 6 proton, 6 neutrons, 6 electrons = the isotope last forever = the sane are all about living as long as possible, no matter what) which is a trait of one who gets the education and becomes very left brain dominate as opposed to one who is cerebrally focused which is one who applies the remedy after getting the education.- 11:53:21 PM

9/22/2009 9:19:55 AM – Right brain is very good at dealing with or detecting paradox. This means left brain is not good at dealing with paradox. A paradox is a proposition that seems contradictory or absurd but in reality expresses a possible truth. What this means is a person who has unveiled right brain may make comments that appear crazy to a person who has not or to a person who has the education and is in extreme left brain and in turn has right brain veiled. This paradox should seem crazy to a person in left brain extreme. The way to life is death.

That is extremely contradictory but it is truth. In order to break the left brain conditioning and reach sound mind(life) or return to harmony which is 50/50 left and right brain one has to defeat their fear of death and that means they have to experience death mindfully. So the way to life is death. So that is a contradictory statement that is absolutely true. One on the left may suggest that is crazy but it is in fact truth. The problem is that comment is complex and right brain deals with complexity and so left brain deals with simplemindedness so one on the left would have trouble grasping that comment on face value unless it was explained in detail. After the education one has this false alter ego dominate, left brain state of mind, they have to kill it or trick it into thinking the being has let go of life and that silences this left brain alter ego and then one returns to sound mind and regains mental function or harmony, so the way to mental life is mental death.- 9:27:40 AM

10:55:59 AM – The concept of belief from a religious point of view is the biggest misunderstanding about religion. Belief from a religious point of view has nothing to do with belief in God. Belief from a religious point of view is belief that these sequential inventions called written language, reading and math do alter the mind or the spirit. They are one in the same. Simply put if a person does not believe the tree of knowledge is theses inventions, written language, reading and math, then they are not a believer and they cannot understand the fear not remedy.

If one misses the point of the tree of knowledge story there is no point in reading any further in the ancient texts. If one does not believe they have been put to sleep mentally by this tree of knowledge then they cannot ever possibly apply the remedy because they do not believe they need to apply the remedy, unless by accident. If one misses what the tree of knowledge is they are dead in the water. There is a reason Genesis is the first book and there is a reason they put that tree of knowledge story right up front. If one does not understand that initial story the game is over.

That initial story about the tree of knowledge is the cornerstone of all the text after it. Every sentence in all the ancient texts is relative to that tree of knowledge story. The texts are suggesting, this is what happens if you get the tree of knowledge and do not apply the fear not remedy. So a believer is one who understands what tree of knowledge represents, demotic and math, believes the remedy is fear not, lose your life to preserve it, submit to fear, then one applies the remedy.

If one does not believe it is possible this education put them in a mental state of mind that is in fact unsound then they are beyond help. The complexity of that is that right brain deals with creativity and imagination and thinking out of the box, or considering all possibilities so one who gets the education has a veiled right brain, and so believing is very difficult. It is even more difficult because one in this unsound state of mind also has a very strong ego and they will have trouble admitting they were mentally harmed by the education.

The most difficult aspect of admitting one perhaps was harmed by this education mentally is if one understands that is reality their entire understanding is shattered so they will resist admitting this education in fact harmed them. The reason their entire understanding will be shattered is because of this comment "they know not what they do." One has to look at this comment on the deepest levels because it reveals something that leaves one with only two options and both options are very dark.

[Luke 23:32 And there were also two other, malefactors, led with him to be put to death.

169

Luke 23:33 And when they were come to the place, which is called Calvary, there they crucified him, and the malefactors, one on the right hand, and the other on the left.

Luke 23:34 Then said Jesus, Father, forgive them; for they know not what they do. And they parted his raiment, and cast lots.

Luke 23:35 And the people stood beholding. And the rulers also with them derided him, saying, He saved others; let him save himself, if he be Christ, the chosen of God.]

The word malefactor is an evil doer but that is really explaining a person on the left or the sane because they exhibit mental traits relative to the seven deadly sins because they are of unsound mind or in extreme left brain because of the education conditioning. So this is suggesting these two evildoers so to speak were conditioned with the education and then exhibited behavior that broke the laws of the ones who conditioned them and now they are being killed because of this behavior. So the powers that be conditioned these beings into this unsound state of mind and then when they exhibited behavior which is physical based centeredness they were killed for doing so.

(33) is a code. This is complex because it appears like a minor detail to the sane but it is in fact a trait of a sound mind. One was on his right and one was on his left. This means Jesus was in the middle of the road or in the middle. Sound mind denotes left and right hemispheres are both working 50/50 which is harmony. Right brain has a lot of ambiguity or doubt so one has a normal amount of doubt and that doubt is what allows one to considering many options before making a final judgment on a situation. One of these evil doers so to speak eventually believed Jesus and one did not. Believed as in believed Jesus was not harmful but speaking truth. The deeper meaning is both of these men were getting ready to die and they were looking at death in the eyes and one of them came to his senses or woke up just before he died and one did not.

These men were in a situation similar to the Abraham and Isaac technique they were unable to run from certain death because they were forced into death. These beings were tied to a cross and were going to be killed so they were mindful of death. This is similar to a person with a terminal illness and towards the end they suggest "I have made my peace". What that really means is they have left go of life which is physical existence. They have their physical affairs in order so to speak. Once a person makes peace with letting go of the physical they in turn increase their cerebral awareness.

[John 3:30 He must increase, but I must decrease.]

This is the scale of weight. As one side goes up one side goes down. There are a few ways to look at this. As one holds unto the material things more the cerebral things diminish. As one holds on to physical life more and more the cerebral things diminish. This is of course relative to ones who have not applied the remedy to the full measure.

Once the fear not remedy is applied one is going into the cerebral no matter what they do. The comment that money has no power over me simply means one has applied the remedy and they are no longer physical or materialistically focused. The mind itself will not become excited over a stack of gold, is one way to look at it. A mind in this cerebral state is more concerned with cerebral aspects so it can no longer crave physical or materialistic aspects. It is not a person is so good because they are not materialistic it is the mind itself no longer is drawn to these material aspects like it was before the remedy is applied. That means the materialism is a symptom of an unsound mind or a symptom of the neurosis the education causes. The reason for that is because once the fear not remedy is applied one cannot take it back or go back.

It is easier to look at it like one is born and then they get the education and then they apply the remedy and then they go back to sound mind. That is why one cannot go back after they apply the remedy because they negate the damage done by the left brain conditioning and revert to sound mind and there is nothing to go back from. So the heightened awareness and telepathy and feeling through vision and extreme concentration is normal, and if one does not have those they are mentally of unsound mind.

So the education robs a person mentally of what is theirs to begin with so it makes one mentally retarded as in hindered, because they are never told the remedy to the education, so they are left with half a mind and left to deal with life with half a mind, and so they are abused or tortured because they have one hand tied behind their back. It is actually much worse than that because of this next line.

[Luke 23:34 Then said Jesus, Father, forgive them; for they know not what they do. And they parted his raiment, and cast lots.]

First off Jesus is saying Father you forgive them because I do not. That may come as a shock to the sane but the reality is the sane do not know what they do or say. This comes down to the only two possible options. Both options are very dark. If a person knows not what they do they are either insane or possessed. If a person educates a child into this left brain state and a society gives money to encourage this conditioning of other children into this left brain state, and in turn robs these children of their minds because the society does not suggest the fear not remedy, then the entire society is a mental rapist of children's minds and does not even know that is what they do, so they are either totally insane or possessed by a sinister dark aspect.

No matter what the option in reality is these beings conditioned into this state of mind have no business being allowed around children, being able to pass laws, being able to wage wars being in possession of weapons and most of all they should not be in a situation to judge others because they are either insane or possessed.

This comment at the end of that line [And they parted his raiment, and cast lots.] is a symptom of one who is conditioned into the extreme left. They are gambling for his garments. Garments are physical or materialistic aspects. So Jesus is saying forgive them for they know not what they do, and then they are showing what they do which is they are materialistically focused which means they are of unsound mind because they are killing the one being that can wake them up and holds the keys, which is "fear not" to break their neurosis, and all they can do is think about material objects.

These people are not killing Jesus as much as they are dooming their self to a long life of mental sorrow. The sane killed Jesus, killed Mohammed, killed Socrates, killed Buddha and a host of others and then the sane walk around and have no clue they just hung their self

172

because only these beings held the key to break the neurosis which is fear not.

So it all comes down to one question. Why are the righteous always getting slaughtered shouldn't the insane or possessed be getting slaughtered? Shouldn't the ones who mentally rape children and mentally rape everyone by force of law be getting slaughtered? Why are the ones who are trying to assist others to revert back to sound mind after the education getting slaughtered? Perhaps those questions are light years beyond the abominations mental ability to ever understand.

[Luke 23:35 And the people stood beholding. And the rulers also with them derided him, saying, He saved others; let him save himself, if he be Christ, the chosen of God.]

So the sane are sitting here killing this wise being who can assist them to revert back to sound mind and they mock him. This is the trend of the sane. They are a threat to everything they touch. The greatest right the sane will ever have is to be put in a cage and kept away from children and others so they do not infect them. That is the only right the sane will ever have.

The sane are not going to apply fear not because they are too stupid to understand they need to.

Only the suicidal have a chance to wake up and they are the meek because they do not deem their self(left brain alter ego) as important enough to live. All the other sane are not worth the paper money they pray to. Perhaps civilization is going to have to redefine the words depth, understanding, wisdom, intelligence and God because I understand they define the word darkness quite well. - 12:09:25 PM

Moments of clarity can be harsh.
Si EGO necessarius an exercitus EGO would have unus.

5:20:31 PM - They ask questions that are meaningless and come to conclusions based on their meaningless questions. They have no eyes.

So you go out and keep destroying children's mind with your wisdom invention because I am going to sit here and remind you of your fruits until kingdom come.

These are our fruits.

J. N. (18) committed suicide by hanging at his home
A. T. (18) allegedly committed suicide by an unknown method
A. F. (23) committed suicide by gunshot wound to the head
C. E. (16) allegedly committed suicide by hanging
S. M. (14) allegedly committed suicide by hanging

These are our fruits because of the invention, our wise education.

Those who lose their life will preserve it. [Luke 17:33 Whosoever shall seek to save his life shall lose it;] [John 12:25 He that loveth his life shall lose it;]. Only the suicidal understand the definition of meek everyone else is in various stages of arrogance and what's funny about that is all of the sane are suicidal. The sane will kill their own children over a penny.

The sane are unable to function without their material things and that is their Achilles heel. Take the money away from the sane and they will destroy their self trying to get it back. The sane keep conditioning the children to be like them and that is why they are their own worst enemy. The sane kill their only hope and so they kill their self and so they are death. The sane are the viper that bites itself. They are the very nature of the darkness because the darkness is unto itself physical death. The cycle of the sane is self sustaining destruction and the end result is death. There is no possible way the sane can avoid their own eventual destruction because everything they do only leads to death and that is what the curse is.

The sane cannot break the curse and apply fear not because they are too afraid. The sane have to not be afraid to apply the remedy but they are too afraid. This means the curse is unbreakable except once in a while someone breaks it by accident. Only an accident can break the curse because the curse is unbreakable otherwise. The curse itself is airtight but once in a while an accident breaks the curse so there is no way to break the curse on purpose. One may perceive they break the curse with intentional methods but they are just kidding their self. One has to believe they are dead set on killing their self and then by some miracle they go all the way but still fail. That is an indication of how strong the curse is.

[Luke 17:33 - and whosoever shall lose his life shall preserve it.] This is not a joke or a comedy routine. This is saying you are doomed. Doomed means you are cursed forever and ever. You just keep telling yourself you are just fine and you love life and love everything around you because you are so doomed that is the only way you can remain breathing. The ones you trust, your peers and your parents and the adults you trusted as a child cursed you into infinitely and you cannot even break that curse, you can only hope to slightly reduce that curse. Simply put you do not have the fortitude the suicidal have. You mock the suicidal but I assure you they have more fortitude than you will ever be able to ever imagine ever.

The next time you hear about someone who is suicidal you go and wash their feet with your hair and you tell them you wish you had the fortitude they have. You ask them why God gave them so much fortitude and yet cursed you with arrogance. You ask them what the definition of meek is because you have no clue. And I can leave that in my poorly disguised dairy because you cannot understand anything I say ever.- 5:49:36 PM

11:43:22 PM – [Exodus 32:19 And it came to pass, as soon as he came nigh unto the camp, that he saw the calf, and the dancing: and Moses' anger waxed hot, and he cast the tables out of his hands, and brake them beneath the mount.]

I blame everything I have written up to this point and will ever write on anger waxing, So now matter what I ever say you just tell yourself its anger waxing because I am not deleting one sentence for your sake. - 11:44:57 PM

The greatest fool is the one who tells jokes because he cannot understand wisdom.

9/23/2009 1:07:06 PM –
"A church is a hospital for sinners, not a museum for saints."

Abigail Van Buren

Religion is there to assist one with applying the fear not remedy, not a place to idolize those who have applied it.

"Where there is charity and wisdom, there is neither fear nor ignorance."

Francis of Assisi

When fear is gone the proper traits replace it.

"It is not fitting, when one is in God's service, to have a gloomy face or a chilling look."

Francis of Assisi

When it's spear of mocking pierces deep do not let it see you weep.
When Maya gets angry that means you are winning.
When in person look it in the eyes so it will be unable to devise.

This of course needs clarification. Once one break's the curse they are in neutral this means they are a mimic to those they are around relative to their mindset. One can go into a chat room with a good positive mindset and then suggest the remedy and then be attacked and then one becomes violent mentally. This is because one is nothing or in nothingness so one mimics whoever they are around. This is similar to how a child can mimic those they are around. This is also why certain ones in nothingness hang around each other in Temples and do not mingle often with the world as it were. This is also why some monks in the Western religions have communes and they allow the sane to come to them, but they do not go out among the sane. This mimic state of mind means one can read the mind of the ones they speak to and also get the spirit of what the sane say and they can tell who they are dealing with, so one become combative. In person is it different because one has heightened awareness so one can get that feeling of perfection from vision from the sane, and use that to keep them clam when they speak to the sane.

It is not about one being insulted by the words when the sane mock them it is more about detecting the violent tendencies of the sane and then being prone to mimic them. This is why many who are awake to a degree hide away. They hide away because when they are around the sane they read the violent tendencies of the sane and become violent mentally.

The sane thrive on the pack mentality this is why they are sheep. One will mock you and then another will mock you and then many will jump on that band wagon and this is why the wise ones, like the disciples where killed because the pack detects this being that is unlike their pack so they kill it. The pack does not like outsiders, would be a good way to look at it.

Some try to disguise the comments by suggesting psychology or how the brain works and this is because the sane who are religious cannot be taught their religion because they misunderstand their own religion, so one comes across as a heretic. The problem with that is religious people know little about the mind or how the brain even works or about psychology. This is a symptom they are so far to the left brain they only see parts. They cannot make the connection that mind is spirit and spirit is mind so psychology is relative to spirit and so mind is also relative to spirit. They believe there is a soul but it cannot be their mind.

The meek, depressed, are the best ones to speak to because they are in a mental state of humility. That does not mean you are going to win, and considering the sane keep pumping out new sane with their slave making machine called education it all comes back to the fact, pick anyone you want.

I do not detect the Abraham and Isaac technique which is mental suicide is going to go over well with any of them. They have to understand something is wrong first and if they do not then they have no reason to apply the remedy. Suggesting to someone with a strong sense of time, hunger and strong emotions which is a symptom of the neurosis, doesn't work because they are surrounded by ones who have all those symptoms. This is also the pack mentality. Everyone they know has the education so everyone they know is in neurosis

177

so they perceive they are normal traits. That a good indication of the impossibility of turning the tide on this neurosis.

Suggesting an unpopular truth is difficult and suggesting an illusion shattering truth is nearly impossible. First off the sane do not like change and that is because left brain likes safety and is not very good at adaptation so to suggest to them they need to change is not going to be accepted. Secondly they have to defeat their fear of death and their Hypothalamus is not working properly so they are very prone to fear so that aspect isn't going to go over well. This is why Adam suggested do not even eat off that tree. Once one eats off the tree they are going to have mental effects that they may never be able to remedy. Is a person's mind worth less than getting this education? It is simply an either or. If you get this education and do not get any fear not conditioning you end up with no mind so what is even the point of the education except to make many brain dead people swiftly that are prone to fear and are nervous wrecks.

What is the point of the education since when you put one through all those years of left brain conditioning they come out mentally hindered which is what retardation is. Why are we taking a being that is mentally fine and then ruining it with this left brain sequential conditioning called education? Fixing something that is not broken is insanity because one is hallucinating that something is broken which is why they determine it needs fixing to begin with. Of course that kind of thinking is far too complex for the sane because all they have to ponder that with is their elementary pinprick sequential logic. So it all really comes down to one comment.

[Ecclesiastes 3:8 - A time to love, and a time to hate; a time of war, and a time of peace.]

So I nearly killed myself and accidentally lost my fear, and then woke up to this unnamable mental power that enables me to figure out how I was put to sleep, and then this unnamable mental power enables me to figure out many are also put to sleep, and I am suppose to have humility and compassion even when the unnamable mental power keeps reminding me "They are doing what they did to you to children and others right now as you slothfully sit here and spit out words that will never solve the problem."

I hope for the sake of the sane I accidentally applied fear not and got infinitely dumb because if I did not there is going to be a Red Sea. I already know what there is going to be, so why don't you try to use your pinprick sequential logic and figure out why I know what there is going to be. The time for peace and blindness has passed. I need all the filler I can get. I almost gave up on books last night and then I reminded myself I am not even trying yet.- 2:43:00 PM

3:43:28 PM – I submit I come across very arrogant, self centered and condescending but the deeper reality is I accidentally applied this ancient fear not aspect and my mental capacity went through the roof and my left brain keeps telling me things I cannot do and my right brain keeps proving that is wrong. The right brain seeks out problems that have no solution just so it can have a goal that will keep it thinking and pondering and ticking away.

Think about a person who is paralyzed their whole life and then one day they can walk and they go on a long walk and they walk all the time and it is not about where they walk it is just they want to walk. So I have found this impossible mission. I have found that I cannot wake up anyone like I woke up and that is great news to the right brain because it has a lot to ponder and think about and many strategies to consider in this impossible mission. So I am self centered in relation to I am seeking this impossible mission as a way to keep testing the limits of this right brain I accidentally unveiled.

This is the strange thing about the right brain. It is not concerned with winning or losing it just wants to keep thinking. Trying to communicate with one in extreme left brain when I have right brain active is impossible. If it is not impossible I do not want to know it's not impossible. I want to get all the mileage I can out of this right brain while I can. Solving a problem is very limiting. If I think everything is fine I am not going to have much to think about. Luxury is sloth and urgency requires thinking. Relative to the problems this left brain education creates in society as whole I figured it out and there is no question in my mind I have figured it out but that is bad news because I defeated that aspect so now I have to find more things to defeat mentally or things to ponder. This is why I am selfish because I am not trying to really help anyone I am trying to find a problem this right brain cannot solve.

This right brain allowed me to solve the greatest mystery of all of civilization in nine months and the problem is now that I solved that I have to find a greater problem and that greater problem is convincing the ones on the left that my solving of this great mystery is true and that is an impossible mission and that is what right brain loves.

I am creating this me against everything mentality in my head because right brain will not have it any other way. That is contrary to left brain. Left brain likes strength in numbers and that is what the herd mentality is all about so right brain likes the hardest route and that is the solo route. In relation to how many people have been conditioned into this extreme left brain and how many are still being conditioned our fate as a species is certainly sealed so there is no real point to why I would try to unseal our fate as a species when I understand that fate is sealed, but that is the goal and an impossible goal at that. I accidentally unveiled right brain and it wants the hardest challenge in the universe and it doesn't want any help and it doesn't want to even win, it just wants something to challenge it.

So right brain is unnamable because it ways go against all the ways and logic of left brain. Right brain is the machine and the machine seeks impossibility because impossibility allows the machine to test itself. This is all done on the cerebral level so physically I don't need to leave my isolation chamber to wage war against impossibility. The deeper reality is right brain is so powerful one does not even sense fatigue or stress even when dealing with an impossible challenge. That is relative to fear creating panic and panic creates stress and stress creates missteps so when fear is gone panic and stress are also gone. I am not warmed up so at times I forget who is on my side. I forget right brain cannot be defeated at anything. There is nothing right brain cannot ponder itself through in short order but I am not use to that so at times I have doubts about that.

That is expected because one who is in the extreme left brain for so long as in a life time and then unveils this powerhouse tends to try to think how they use to think and they just need to get use to this unnamable power house called right brain. Right brain is too powerful so that may be why we subconsciously invented something that would veil it.

As a species maybe we invented something that would dumb us down to make life a challenge. Simply put we have huge brains and life was way too easy and so we made this invention and now life is not way too easy. That is a clue as to how powerful right brain is once it is unveiled. So as a species we were so smart we actually wanted to become dumber and maybe we became too dumb in this effort. So we invented written language and understood it would veil the right brain and make us dumber but it made us way dumber. That could be what it is. We were Gods mentally and we wanted to make life a bigger challenge and that is right brain thinking, wanting impossibility and so that what we got and now, life is very difficult and we are destor6ying everything and fighting each other and we have lots of challenges we can never win against and that is perhaps exactly what we wanted.

Right brain wants conflict and problems cerebrally because it's so powerful it can do the impossible and solve the impossible problems effortlessly. What would you do if you could solve every single problem there is in nine months? You would seek out more problems to solve but you would not find any so you wouldn't want to solve every problem there is because then right brain would be out of work.

Perhaps this line of comments is too deep for some. - 4:22:07 PM

Perhaps one day they will build a robot with a brain that can emulate the brain or mind of one who has been conditioned into extreme left brain but they will need a robot brain the size of the universe to emulate right brain.

You ignore idiots who suggest the amount of money you have determines your intelligence. You ignore idiots who suggest your education level determines your intelligence. You ignore those idiots because their very own words prove they are idiots.

9/24/2009 5:43:29 PM – I give up. I cannot win. I quit. - 5:43:47 PM

7:40:13 PM – I am back for more punishment. This is in relation to how this left brain state of mind causes one to bring harm to their self without that said person being aware of it. I am using extremes to make the point. The food supply is actually the cause of much crime and killings. If a producer of food charges for food and the only people that can get that food are ones who slave for it then there is always going to be ones who cannot afford that food and so they go hungry. Then they are forced to ask for food and that places a burden on social programs that give away food or food stamps.

Some people do not want to be reduced to this perceived low class of asking for food stamps so they may resort to crime. They are forced to resort to crime because civilization as it is has destroyed all the free food sources. Simply put one is not able to go hunt and gather. Civilization has partitioned all the land and sold it off and then paved over what is left so one is bound to subscribe to the ones who produce and sell food for money. So the complexity is we have destroyed all the free food sources and now we are a slave to ones who produce food. Certainly one can go live in the wilderness but first they have to buy that land or they are trespassing and are illegal and will be thrown in jail. We have done this to ourselves and we are having all these troubles and because we are of unsound mind we come up with stupid solutions. We lock people in cages who steal to get something to eat because we have destroyed all the free food they should be able to get to begin with. This is an indication that this left brain sequential mental state leaves one not being able to think clearly. It leaves one shooting their self in the foot while thinking that will help them walk. When the mind is ruined one will only be left with ruins. - 7:50:49 PM

10:38:56 PM – Dawn your snorkels.
Hypothalamus - activates "fight or flight" response
Amygdala - decodes emotions; determines possible threat; stores fear memories

Point: Twelve years of left brain sequential education alters the mind into an extreme left brain state.

Point: This extreme left brain state creates a mind in disharmony and so parts of the brain do not act as they should.

Point : The Hypothalamus gives off false signals of fear of words, pictures and ghosts that it should not be giving off if the mind was sound or in harmony.

Point: The Amygdala creates very strong emotions such as depression, fear, sense of loss, insecurity and a host of other signals that are given off as a result of this unsound extreme left brain mental state caused by the years of sequential education.

Point: All these factors combined create a mental state of confusion because these are false signals going through the mind and they hinder one's ability to concentrate and make logical decisions.

[Luke 9:60 Jesus said unto him, Let the dead bury their dead:...]

Let the dead bury their dead denotes the ones who are in this extreme left brain state are simply way to emotional and way to sentimental because this Amygdala is telling them to be depressed over a dead person even when they fully understand everyone must die eventually. The sane at times kill their self because someone they knew dies because their emotions are false because this Amygdala is not working properly because their mind is conditioned so far to the left none of these parts in the brain that are physiologically undamaged simply not working properly because the mind itself is unbalanced from twelve years of sequential left brain conditioning called education.

So the education itself is far more damaging to the mind than anything known to man because it is taught by people with unsound minds who are not even aware of what kind of damage twelve years of hardcore sequential left brain conditioning can do to the mind if not properly administered. Simply put the educators do not know what kind of damage they are doing to people so they do it and then suggest they are wise in doing it.

A person loses their job. The hypothalamus sends them a signal they should be afraid because they lost their ability to make money and now they are doomed because they won't have any food. The Amygdala gives false emotional signals and that person starts to think their employer fired them for spite and so that person determines they need to get payback and so they make some rash decision to exact their revenge.

A person eats to much because the Amygdala keeps telling them they are hungry every hour on the hour. It keeps telling a drug user they need drugs every hour on the hour. It tells a person whatever they have to do to make money is good because that money will make them feel good. It tells a person to drive 90 miles an hour because that will make them have fun and feel good. It tells a country it has been insulted by another country and so that initial country must wage war to restore its pride. It tells a civilization to pave over the wildlife so it will feel safe. It tells the world to condition the children into this same left brain state of mind so the children will be wise and thus safe.

The point is as a society, we are altering the mind with this sequential heavy education and twelve years of it to boot and when one plays around with the mind that is in perfect harmony to begin with at birth the only thing they are going to end up with is a mental abomination and that is what society is. We destroyed ourselves because we thought we were smart enough to alter the mind, because we assumed it was not in perfect harmony at birth and we were mistaken. We as a species made one miscalculation, that miscalculation was that we assumed nature or God or whatever you want to call it made a mistake in creating our minds and that miscalculation cost us everything. Don't you ever tell me everything is going to be just fine, you save that speech for the children you mentally rape on a daily basis.- 11:13:03 PM

Vanity - http://www.youtube.com/watch?v=4nIhvhnW1lI
I don't try because you can't even break the curse.

[Genesis 3:17 ..., and hast eaten of the tree, of which I commanded thee, saying, Thou shalt not eat of it: cursed is the ground for thy sake; in sorrow shalt thou eat of it all the days of thy life;]

Somehow I broke the curse but you can't. There is not one single human being I have talked to that has even attempted to apply fear not and the ones who are "awake" that I have spoken to do not even know what the tree of knowledge even is, so they are not awake either. If I tell you I am the only human being who was cursed and then broke the curse you will call me egotistical and if I tell you that you can break this curse, I call Adam a liar.

[Genesis 3:17 ..., cursed is the ground for thy sake; in sorrow shalt thou eat of it all the days of thy life;]

I am an accident that should not have happened and the only ones who have a light chance of having the accident are suicidal people and they have to be very dumb in their attempt at suicide to go the full measure and fully break the curse. And so I will tell you the very fact I am in infinity with no sense of time means I am forced to try to suggest this remedy to people even while I know fully they cannot break the curse so I tell you, I am doomed to vanity. When engaged in infinite vanity filler is important. Talk about moments of doubt. - 11:29:30 PM

Do you really think if I say everything properly and act properly and spell all the words properly that is going to get a person who loves "life" to mentally let go of it? This is why the emotional addiction these ill functioning parts of the brain, the Amygdala and Hypothalamus, create are far stronger than any argument I can ever make. The sane listen to their heart or their intuition and their heart or intuition is a liar or sending them false signals so I assure you I write in diary format because even early on after the accident I knew I stood no chance. I write in diary format because I no longer talk to you because I don't talk to cursed people because they are cursed and [Genesis 3:17 ..., in sorrow ... all the days of thy life;]. I can't trust the dust. - 11:38:45 PM

To clarify. [Genesis 3:24 So he drove out the man; and he placed at the east of the garden of Eden Cherubims, and a flaming sword which turned every way, to keep the way of the tree of life.]

Once one gets the education they get thrown out of the Garden of Life and get thrown into Cherebims. That word means imaginary which is a nice way to say hallucination world, it's an imaginary figure or an imaginary life. You are in fact in a dream world which means you are asleep and everything you think is real is not real. Your mind is hallucinating and perhaps everything you think is important is not important. Every decision you think is wise is foolish. Everything you think is safe is unsafe. You are in a reverse alternate reality. You think it is unsafe to face your fear of death but that is the only way you can escape so you can never escape because you see the way out as a dangerous proposition. You see the door out of the reverse alternate world as a demon you must run from, but in reality you must run to that thing that scares you in order to get out of that door and back into reality.

Your mind keeps telling you to run away from the exit door that leads you out of the hallucination world you are trapped in. Perhaps you simply love the hallucination world you live in too much. Perhaps you love what you perceive is life in the reverse reality you are trapped in. Maybe all those things you love about what you perceive is life are carefully crafted desires and cravings to keep you trapped in that reverse reality. Do you think Jesus was kidding when he said this?

[John 12:25 - He that loveth his life shall lose it;].

Mental suicide might cost you what you perceive is life and that is a price you are not willing to pay because you love this perceived life because it has so many nice perks. You would rather not risk losing all those perks you perceive in your reverse reality hallucination world. I am telling you to your face you are in an alternate reality and you were put there by the ones you trusted by way of the education system conditioning. None of that is even important and those details are not even important because the truth is I do not believe anyone can get out once they get sent there except by accident. Once one gets the education they are stuck in that hallucination world.
[Psalms 37:22 - For such as be blessed of him shall inherit the earth; and they that be cursed of him shall be cut off.]

They certainly throw around the word cursed a lot in these ancient texts someone should scold them. Don't go around telling people they are cursed cause they don't want to know they are cursed. I certainly would never publish a book and suggest six billion people are cursed, imagine the consequences. The words "cut off" denotes the cursed are put into this hallucination reverse reality.

[Genesis 3:24 So he drove out the man; and he placed at the east of the garden of Eden Cherubims, and a flaming sword which turned every way, to keep the way of the tree of life.]

"he placed" and "cut off" are the same thing. So the sane are opt in this Garden of Imaginary reality. They go around and say things like "I will kill a herd of buffalo for 50 bucks because I am wise.", "I will destroy and entire forest to build a condominium that no one will ever live in because I am wise." They will say "I will ensure my own first born child is given the education and curse them to the reality I have been cursed to, because I am wise."

My point is something had mercy on me and said "Any idiot that fails at suicide 30 times in 10 years automatically gets a ticket to ride out of the alternate reality hallucination world."

I do not even remember what fear is like anymore at this stage so certainly I am not afraid to tell you what I understand. I submit this is the worst of the 10 books I have written so far but before I get to the 20th book this book will seem like a wonderful thing. The further I go into the progression the further I get away from that hallucination world and so the harder it is for me to communicate with you.

I am going into the garden in a chariot and I cannot slow it down. I cannot even convince the ones who know me about the merits of fear not so I certainly cannot convince you of it. All I can say is I understand what these wise beings were saying and I will try to keep communicating with you as long as I can. If I fail I fail like all the others have and that's okay because I am a failure. That's what they said I was when I failed a 50 rule comma test and could not get into college as a result so they said "You are a failure." And so I failed at suicide 30 times because I thought I was a failure and that is exactly what I had to be in order to break free of that alternate imaginary reality I was trapped in.

So being a failure and being meek is the key to escape. What you think is wrong is really right in your hallucination alternate reality. You don't want to go to that scary dark cemetery alone at night, do it. You don't want to turn off the lights after that scary movie, do it. You don't want to listen to certain music, do it. You don't want to say certain bad words, do it. You don't want to go to certain evil chat rooms, do it. You don't want to mentally let go of life, do it. You don't want to let go of your luxuries, do it. You have to start thinking in reverse or you will never escape that anti-world you are in would be the point of this lesson.- 12:34:03 AM

Once there was a man who fell upon the sand,
He could not understand I offered up my hand.

He said the sand was warm and said the sand was nice.
He said the sand was warm not once, not twice, but thrice.

Little did he know the sand was not so nice.
I offered up my hand not once, not twice, but thrice.

Just before his hand was covered in the sand,
I asked him for my name, he did not understand.

I could see his eyes sinking in the sand.
I use to know his name and offered him my hand, not once, not twice, but thrice.

Now I stay away, out far at sea.
The inviting shore, I can hardly see.
The sand is warm there, the sand is nice, a man once told me, not once, not twice, but thrice.

3:23:26 AM – I am aware I sound rather defeated at times but that is actually a symptom of the ambiguity or doubt in right brain once it is unveiled. I am not doubting little petty things I am doubting this battle can be won because it is so deep and so complicated the right brain keeps me humble when it suggests I cannot convince anyone of these things I speak of and that allows me to ponder further and come to further methods to communicate.

The ambiguity in right brain keeps one honest in respect to it keeps one questioning their methods and that leads to an ever refined method. Right brain is like a sifter. One throws in all this data and little aspects of that data start sifting out. If one lays out everything I have written there will be lots of contradictions because they are really notes. The ideals or cerebral concepts lead to many branches and some branches lead to other branches and some branches are dead ends. This is why the right brain has a short term memory and has a good long term memory. I keep little parts from each conversation I have with the ones in chat rooms and I tag mentally the parts that work and the parts that don't and that is the same with conversations in general.

Some things stick out and are put in long term memory and some things are simply forgotten. This is suggesting how complex this machine called right brain is once unveiled and you have one also so I am not pushing my own buttons. It is a powerhouse that cannot even be explained so unnamable is the only possible explanation. In all reality I am on a train and I am not really driving the train but I am pleased with the scenery that goes by. I see a pretty tree but it goes by so fast I cannot focus on that pretty tree because a pretty lake is now in view, and then a pretty mountain is in view the next moment. So one gets the impression they are experiencing nothingness but in reality the machine is processing information so fast one does not even have time to remain in one state of mind for very long. I do not really think people are bad I think the machine has been veiled because of the education and I simply try to suggest ways to turn it back on. I think if we can at least look at the sequential education aspect we can come up with some techniques to reduce the unwanted mental side effects of the education.

There are some patterns I have been pondering and these are just patterns and not statements about anything. The people who found Buddha's teaching memorized them all. The pattern there is massive long term memorization. The Madrasah is simply a place of learning but one strategy is they make a student memorize a long text in full. This is not memorizing a page this is memorizing a novel or two. That appears to me to be a right brain conditioning aspect and contrary to that is short term memorization which is like traditional education in the West. Short term memory tests, even a midterm test is short term memory because one crams for it at the last moment and after the test they pretty much forget everything. One cannot fake memorizing a novel or two, word for word.

I am stuck on the fence about whether this is not just a psychological misunderstanding or something on the sinister side, so to speak. Perhaps I take for granted this conditioning has been going on for 5000 years or more now. My sense of time is gone so perhaps I do not appreciate that. I am pleased to stay in the frame of mind that it is simple logic that if one does too much sequential left brain conditioning they will have unbalanced mind and so we can adjust and remedy that and no one is to blame and everything can be worked out. Perhaps that is my wishful thinking and thus perhaps my greatest delusion. - 4:00:21 AM

9/25/2009 4:06:30 PM – Here I am pondering. My right brain keeps formulating calculations and its keeps coming back with the fact the sane are too great in number. The sane cannot be stopped and cannot be reasoned with. I look at my tears of frustration as method to formulate a battle plan against the sane. There is nothing in this battle that can defeat me but me because the sane are great in number but they have no chance. The sane have no mind so they cannot compete with a mind. The sane are just a never mind. I will not leave my isolation chamber because after I defeat the sane I do not want anyone to ever say "He had to try."- 4:18:35 PM

10:01:19 PM – We have such large powerful brains we could not even tell how powerful we were so we decided to try to get powerful because we were so intelligent with these large powerful brain we could not even tell how powerful we were, and in the process of trying to get more powerful we made ourselves dumb.

So now we are trying to figure out who is most intelligent because we do not even realize we are all so intelligent we cannot even figure out how intelligent we are. We invent the word intelligent and then try to fit ourselves into that word but we are far beyond the definition of intelligent so we keep dumbing ourselves down to fit into this narrow definition of intelligent. Whatever intelligent is we are far beyond that definition so we have to invent ways to become dumb so we can live up to this narrow minded definition called intelligence. These huge brains we have are so powerful we lose ourselves in our own vast intelligence and then we get trapped because we are beyond our own ability to even understand.

Once in a while someone wakes up and finds out how intelligent we really are and tries to explain it but the words can never explain it so they end up failing to explain it properly. They try to say God and try to say unnamable and try to say beyond understanding but those words also do not explain it, they all fall short of explaining what these huge brains we have are capable of. Our vast intelligence caused by these huge brains lead us into trouble at times. We try to make life difficult because life is so effortless for ones with such huge brains there is no reason we shouldn't make life hard.

This is all relative to becoming lost in our own beyond understanding intelligence. If we struggle that's fine and if we do not that's fine. We cannot escape our huge brains and our unnamable intelligence. We are so intelligent we cannot even understand it so we actually trick ourselves into seeing mountains because the flat ground is far too simple. We try to compensate this unnamable intelligence by throwing up road blocks just to give us something to do. We try to get wiser and at the same time through this left brain education make ourselves dumber. We are in fact doing lost of things to accomplish nothing but that is not important because we still cannot escape these huge brains we have.

We create problems then we try to solve them and then we create more problems with that solution. Nothing else is really happening but simply digging a hole, falling it, climbing out only to fall in it again. One cannot escape their brain and the brain in humans is way too big so we had to find a way to turn the brain down so life would be a challenge. It's like a video game where you have all the cheat codes and you have unlimited money and unlimited lives and you can never lose no matter what and so that game gets very boring and pointless. So then you turn off the cheat codes and the game is a challenge again and the game is real again. The turning off of the cheat codes or turning down the brains unnamable power creates drama. "You might lose the game now." Life with these huge brains we have is exactly like shooting fish in a barrel, it is boring. We are supreme beings that are bored out of our minds and so we turn the mind power setting down to about level one and then we have this uncertainty again.

Think about all the conflicts in the world. Country against country and ideals against ideals. No country is better and no ideal is better but they do make a nice platform for conflict and that conflict creates drama and that drama eases the boredom. This is what vanity is. We have these huge brains and everything is total boredom unless we turn our brains off.

If we were trying to win and trying to get smarter we would condition our brain to the right hemisphere because that is the complex hemisphere that operates in random access and that is the powerhouse but in reality we condition our minds into the sequential simple minded hemisphere which is left brain and so we are in reality making ourselves dumber so life will be a challenge. That is what we have to do because our brains are abnormally huge.

When one is in a infinity state of mind or no sense of time they simply are so cerebral the physical world is not even considered. One still eats food but they never are hungry so they don't eat much. One cannot be satisfied by money or land or material things so they are all meaningless. One is so cerebral all of the material things just fade away. One can have anything they desire in the cerebral world so there is no point in fighting over material things. These huge brains when they are full power are so intelligent they do not even acknowledge physical gain on any level at all. The mind at full power is not afraid of death because it already understands what death is. The mind at full power already understands everything about everything. This is why we had to dumb ourselves down because all mystery was gone.

There was no such thing as mystery to anyone. No person knew more than any other person because everyone knew everything about everything. This may seem impossible but the reality remains. We are in fact conditioning ourselves into the retarded hemisphere of the brain and it is considered normal and it is accepted worldwide and it is encouraged and even forced by law that one is conditioned into the retarded hemisphere of the brain. This is a logical solution to the problem we are vastly to intelligent with these huge brains.

One gets the education and then they spend the rest of their life trying to achieve full brain function again, and what that gives a person is purpose. So the purpose of conditioning everyone to this left brain state is to give a person purpose so they can try to get back to the state of mind where they have no purpose. This again is vanity. The brain at full power knows everything about everything so there is no purpose to anything so the solution is to turn that down so the more it is turned down the more purpose one has.

This is a natural solution to the problem our brains and thus our minds are way too powerful. We choose purpose over no purpose so we can get back to having no purpose and this means nothing is happening and that is what E=Mc2 is. Nothing is happening, just various states of existence that are in reality all the exact same state.

You know we could not have survived for hundreds of thousands of year in this mental state we are today. We are dumber than we use to be because life was way too easy. I write infinite books because it's too easy to write anything less than infinite books. I will be writing infinite books into infinity and it does not matter if anyone else reads them because I read them. Infinity is vanity.

It is not a question if this fear not remedy will make your life easy the question is what are you going to do when your life is effortless? What are you going to do when you can span an infinite universe in zero seconds? What are you going to do if the most intelligent being in the universe is you? One who has been conditioned into this left brain reality is always trying to make things easier and one who breaks that left brain conditioning is always trying to find a challenge. It is simply a flipped coin. I spend time trying to figure out if I can escape nirvana and some people spend all their money trying to reach nirvana.

I ponder if there is anything I can do to make me dumber and most people spend time trying to figure out ways to get smarter. I pray for ignorance and many pray for wisdom and I am not even warmed up yet. Only a person with half a functioning brain could deduce this huge brain we have could be judged on the merits of a test. This right brain aspect we keep silencing with our wisdom teachings called written language and math is so far beyond a person's ability to even understand that is also beyond a person's ability to even explain or measure. Some people go around and assume there is some intelligent life form in the universe and all we have to do is find them and we will become wise.

We are the only life form in the universe that makes it our goal to make ourselves dumb because we are way too intelligent. Our own intelligence is greater than we are so we dumb this intelligence down and then we can be equal to it. The worst thing you can do is get into the mindset I am special or unique. The reality is you have a brain and all you have to do is condition away this abnormal fear that is a side effect of this left brain conditioning you got a child , forced on your by law, and then you are back to full power. All you have to decide is if you want to float through life or stay down in the trenches.

I wouldn't be too concerned about the fear conditioning no matter I say. You are not really doing anything because it is on a mental level. If anyone ever tells you that you are not intelligent because you did not pass a test or spell a word properly you just remind yourself they are not intelligent because they believe that. One is wise to avoid believing insane people who do not know much to begin with. Some people actually kill their self because some insane person told them they are not intelligent because they did not pass a test created by insane people to determine intelligence.

If you believe insane people they will drive you insane. Insane people go around throwing out judgments about intelligence, even when they understand how huge our brains are, using scales of stupidity. Intelligence is a word someone invented to try to explain something beyond description. I understand many people do not understand they are engaged in vanity. I sit here and wait for October 31st 2009 to get here. That is the one year anniversary since I had the "Ah ha" sensation and everything started making sense. That was about 2 to 5 months since the Abraham and Isaac mental conditioning happened by accident none the less.

I do not even remember the exact date I was laying down after taking a handful of Paxil and my left brain was telling me to run and call for help and my silent right brain said do not call for help let go. I put that left brain in its place forever. It is not even important if I explain these cerebral ideals properly in words. I understand what happened no matter how I put it in words. It is not even important if I can convince one other person in this universe that is what happened because I understand that is what happened.

The reason I am mindful of Oct 31st 2009 is because I sit here trying to explain how powerful right brain is when in reality I have solved everything in less than a year. There is no question about anything ever again relative to human beings and somehow this right brain machine accomplished that in less than one year. I am not aware of what I have done. Somehow this right brain altered the future of mankind forever and even I cannot say that I did it because I am accident. I certainly should feel gratification after such a feat but I feel that would have no purpose. I am not going to stop because the machine is not ready to stop- 11:29:47 PM

9/26/2009 2:00:55 AM – Abraham was wise. Socrates was wise. Buddha was wise. Jesus was wise. Mohammed was wise. You may not agree with all of that but you certainly will agree at least one of those beings was wise. These beings were wise because they all said one similar thing. They all told you how to become wise. This means they were not selfish. They could not become unwise so they tried to explain how everyone could become wise like they were. This denotes lack of ego. They were not holding their wisdom over anyone's head.

[Genesis 15:1 After these things the word of the LORD came unto Abram in a vision, saying, Fear not, Abram: I am thy shield, and thy exceeding great reward.]

So here is where Abraham spilled the beans. He said you apply the fear conditioning and you will get a great reward.

Socrates lived around 469 BCE so he was in sync with Abraham but perhaps Abraham lived before that time period because of this comment.

[Exodus 3:16 Go, and gather the elders of Israel together, and say unto them, The LORD God of your fathers, the God of Abraham, of Isaac, and of Jacob, appeared unto me, saying, I have surely visited you, and seen that which is done to you in Egypt:]

This is a comment by Moses or to Moses whichever way you want to look at it, explaining how Abraham and Isaac came before. The complexity here is Genesis was the first text explaining how to break this curse caused by written language so it is the alpha book relative to this area of the world.

Written language was all over the world at this time and people started breaking that curse and explaining how to break that curse. Socrates was one who broke to curse in Greece.

So Socrates was a big fish in Greece because he broke the curse and he suggested the remedy and he also suggested the youth should perhaps avoid the curse and that is why he was killed.

One of Socrates main points in his teachings was no true Philosopher fears death.

Fear not would include fear of death. If one is facing perceived death and they are told to fear not and they do fear not then they are not afraid of perceived death. Isaac was lying on an alter and Abraham held a knife over him and Isaac did not run so Isaac did not fear death so Isaac applied fear not.

Buddha came along around 563 BCE and he was a big fish that broke the curse in the East. This is not to be confused with they were the only ones who broke the curse but they were the only ones who broke the curse and their writings were recorded and survived and found. I do not know anything about Buddhism but there was one technique I heard of and it fits the pattern.

Sitting alone in a cemetery at night mediating. So one is sitting alone at night in a cemetery and their Hypothalamus says "Run like the wind, ghosts of death are coming" and one does not run like the wind, they fear not and also do not fear death.

The trend in relation to Abraham , Buddha and Socrates is they are simply human beings that that applied this fear not and then that Hypothalamus started working properly again and that also reverted them back to mental harmony or sound mind so they negated this extreme left brain state the written language education put them in. So this sequential education alters the mind to the left and also turns up the Hypothalamus so one is prone to fear and the remedy is to deny the signals of that Hypothalamus and that knocks the mind back into harmony.

Jesus came along 2000 years ago and said this:
[Luke 17:33 Whosoever shall seek to save his life shall lose it; and whosoever shall lose his life shall preserve it.]

He used the word life instead of death. He could have said, whoever shall lose their fear of death preserves it. Or he could have said ,whoever runs from perceived death shall lose it.

Whoever runs from perceived death shall lose it; whoever shall lose their fear of perceived death preserves it.

Isaac did not run from death when he saw that knife over his chest so he preserved it which means he broke the curse or he knocked his mind back into harmony.

Mohammed came about 1500 years ago. He spoke of a Monotheistic faith and he used these names as references Noah,

Moses, Abraham, Jesus. What this proves is he read Genesis and he also read what Jesus said and he agreed with what they said and Mono means one and one denotes wholeness or holistic and that means he simply took what they said and said it a different way. None of the beings in this area of the world could speak about Buddha or Socrates because they didn't even know they existed and visa versa.

Abraham and Isaac story can put all of this together.

What did Isaac do when he saw that knife held over him and perceived his death was imminent?

Fear not. - Abraham

What did Isaac do when he saw that knife held over him and perceived his death was imminent?

No fear of death. - Socrates

What did Isaac do when he saw that knife held over him and perceived his death was imminent?

Not afraid of ghosts or perceived death – Buddha

What did Isaac do when he saw that knife held over him and perceived his death was imminent?

Whosoever shall lose his life shall preserve it. – Jesus

What did Isaac do when he saw that knife held over him and perceived his death was imminent?

Submit (to perceived death). – Mohammed

This is why Mohammed said it is a Monotheistic faith because he was saying exactly what Abraham and Jesus said and also what the other wise beings who woke up in different locations of the earth were saying, the exact same thing and the one common denominator is they all got the written language education, written language was around then and they could write.

There is only one invention at this time that was thought to make you wise and also looked pretty to the eyes.

[Genesis 3:6 And when the woman saw that the tree was good for food, and that it was pleasant to the eyes, and a tree to be desired to make one wise, ...]

There is nothing else at this point in history that could have been thought to make one wise and also look pretty to the eyes but hieroglyphics which is demotic or written language. Adam was not talking about fantasy land he was talking about real things and explaining them in parables. There is no actual tree of knowledge there is only this invention that is thought to make one wise and looks pretty to the eyes and that is written language. It may be pretty to your eyes but it veils your most important eyes and that is your right brain- 2:50:41 AM

4:02:18 AM –

[Genesis 4:1 And Adam knew Eve his wife; and she conceived, and bare Cain, and said, I have gotten a man from the LORD.

Genesis 4:2 And she again bare his brother Abel. And Abel was a keeper of sheep, but Cain was a tiller of the ground.]

[Genesis 11:5 And the LORD came down to see the city and the tower, which the children of men builded.]

This is a good example of how these texts are codes. They are coded so the sane, the ones who are on the left and have not applied the remedy, cannot understand them.

Look at the word man and LORD. A man is a male who gets the education and does not apply the remedy and a LORD is one who gets the education and then applies the remedy which is the same as saying a Master in relation to [Matthew 22:36 Master, which is the great commandment in the law?]

So a LORD is one who has the key or understands the remedy and that name is interchangeable with Master but it is not absolute. Sometimes they say Good Master and Bad Master. [Matthew 19:16 And, behold, one came and said unto him, Good Master, what good thing shall I do, that I may have eternal life?]

199

So a bad master is a taskmaster and one who conditions ones into the left brain state and then turns them into slaves and a good master is one who tries to wake them up or free their mind from the curse using the fear not remedy.

So there is Adam and Eve and Adam is the one who woke up which is why Eve was created from his rib. Created from his rib denotes his struggle or his battle is what enabled Eve to wake up. So from his rib, sacrifice, Eve became, so to speak. But Abraham is the first one to suggest Fear not. This does not mean Adam was the first human being it means Adam was the first to wake up in this area of the world and have his explanations preserved.

So Adam wrote the first few chapters of Genesis and that was his testament or attempt to explain the situation then Abraham came alone perhaps a thousand years later and added on his comments. This is why Mohammed wrote about Adam in the Quran. So Adam was real but the tree of knowledge was symbolism. Abraham figured out the remedy to the tree of knowledge but Adam woke up from the curse but did not call the remedy fear not. Adam suggested sacrifice.

So one gets the education and they enable this left brain extreme state of mind called the alter ego and one must mentally sacrifice that alter ego to revert back to sound mind.

[Gen 4:1…, and bare Cain, and said, I have gotten a man from the LORD.]
So this comment means Adam and Eve had a child that got the education and did not apply the remedy and that is what this line means.

[Genesis 4:2 And she again bare his brother Abel. And Abel was a keeper of sheep, but Cain was a tiller of the ground.]
Abel applied the remedy and he was a keeper of the sheep /flock so he assisted people in waking up but it was not called fear not technique. Cain was a tiller of the ground which means he was of the earth or physically focused which is what a person is when they are in the extreme left brain state.

Cain committed murder and that denotes his fruits and as the world is today the ones conditioned to the left tend to be very militant or violent in contrast to ones who have applied fear not who tend to be very cerebral. So written language was invented around 5400 years ago and so Adam woke up soon after that. So he was one of the first ones to wake up and wrote the first few chapters of the Genesis and then Abraham came along and woke up many years later and he added on to Adams writings. This is the trend of all of these texts.

Adam wakes up and tries his best to explain the curse of the written language then another one wakes up and tries to explain their take, and then another one wakes up and tries to explain their take on the curse. The reality is everyone agrees with Abraham and Adam. Jesus agreed and Mohammed agreed and that is why Monotheistic is suggested because they are all saying one thing just different takes on that one thing, the remedy to the extreme left brain state the written language education leaves one in.

They are rewording the same thing over and over. They are taking the same message and rearranging it in hopes the ones who are in the left brain figure it out. So Abraham woke up and took what Adam said and added "fear not": and also added in a nice fear not technique which is what the Abraham and Isaac story is. The remedy does not change but the ways they explain the remedy changes. One thing is for certain Adam did not live before written language. We know for a fact the aborigines have been around for 50,000 to 60,000 years and the Hindus' have been around for 50,000 years. This is why Adam is the first to wake up from the left brain education relative to that area of the world and has his texts preserved. And the fact Eve says "The LORD gave me a man" denotes Eve bore a child with Adam who got the education and did not apply the remedy and he showed signs of violence which is what his murder of Abel explains. So this was so long ago they may not have been fully aware of the remedy as in ability to explain it like Abraham did.

[Genesis 4:4 And Abel, he also brought of the firstlings of his flock and of the fat thereof. And the LORD had respect unto Abel and to his offering:

Genesis 4:5 But unto Cain and to his offering he had not respect. And Cain was very wroth, and his countenance fell.

201

Genesis 4:6 And the LORD said unto Cain, Why art thou wroth? and why is thy countenance fallen?]

Abel made his offering and this denotes offering as in the offering of Abraham and Isaac. If one faces perceived death and submits to it they sacrifice their self as in their alter ego self which is left brain. So this is saying Abel made his offering and it worked, but Cain did not so he did not apply fear not and he remained in that left brain state of mind. The proof is he had wroth and wroth is wrath, and wrath is anger, and anger is an emotion and a symptom the Amygdala is not working properly because one is mentally conditioned way too far into left brain, because of the sequential based education.

This is why these stories are so difficult to understand because they have to substitute many words to explain things. Why is thy countenance fallen? That is the same as saying a fallen angel. What is a fallen angel? One who gets the education and does not apply the fear not remedy. So LORD means Adam is asking Cain why he is so angry. So Adam has a problem child and he is asking him "Why are you so angry, your brother Abel applied the remedy and I was pleased with his sacrifice but you did not apply the remedy because you are showing signs or anger. That proves you did not apply the remedy so you did not keep the covenant." This is such a long time before even Abraham so it must have been difficult to explain this like we could explain it today. The same definitions but many different words.

This is another way to say anger

[Acts 28:3 And when Paul had gathered a bundle of sticks, and laid them on the fire, there came a viper out of the heat, and fastened on his hand.]

Heat is hot but the anger is so great it comes out of the heat and bites. A hot head is one who is angry. Anger or wrath is because the Amygdala is not working properly. One who has not applied the remedy can lose their temper for hours or days or even weeks and that is impossible to do unless one is in extreme left brain because the mind once the fear is conditioned away will not allow a person to stay in any set state of mind for more than a few minutes simply because right brain ponders so fast, it keeps thoughts moving very fast and in this extreme left brain state thoughts move slowly or are slothful.

Abraham is perhaps the main focus of the west because he not only suggested fear not remedy but he also gave a good example of it, in the Abraham and Isaac explanation. So Adam woke up first and had his word preserved, but Abraham had a very good understanding about the remedy and also how to apply it. So this is why Jesus and Mohammed agreed with Abraham because they read these books and knew Abraham had a very good grasp on the solution, remedy to the curse or the key to the kingdom so to speak.

All of these big fish agreed or were on the same page. These wise beings were all on the same page but the sane are conditioned into the left brain and left brain only see's parts and so they separate these wise beings and create conflicts even when the wise beings all say they all agree.

Jesus agreed Abraham and Mohammed agreed with Jesus and Abraham and if one gets the education and has not applied the covenant, fear not, they can go through their whole life and never see that because they only see things as separate parts.

One gets the education goes extreme left brain and they can only see parts and it is not their fault it is simple reality that left brain see's parts and not wholes. One can never understand this code if they only see parts. So we have these three religions and they are all killing each other because none of them even applied the remedy and so they only see parts when in reality these three religions are all saying the exact same thing, and there is no difference in what these three religions are saying at all but the people who have no applied the remedy can only ever see them as separate parts.

So all the people who fought for these perceived separate belief systems, there is only one word on their head, vanity. The pattern is, although some do understand what fear not means and apply it, the sane eventually forget about it and so the whole cycle starts again. This is the endlessly repeating cycle. Someone wakes up after they get the conditioning and they explain the remedy then time passes and everyone forgets the remedy and then time passes, and someone wakes up and explains the remedy, and this cycle just keeps repeating and has been repeating for perhaps over 5000 years. We are somehow trapped in that cycle. I understand it has a lot to do with control. If everyone had full brain function they would be hard to control because everyone would be as wise as everyone else so no one could be a slave or be taken advantage of. Who is a wise man going to slave for? Once you are conscious you are not going to slave for anyone and that is not good news for the taskmaster. - 5:16:05 AM

I am in another world because all of this makes perfect sense to me and I cannot detect any flaws in how I explain these texts, but sure enough, some of the sane will still say to their buddies "That is not what it says", and we will be doomed to repeat the cycle again and again and again and again and again. - 5:33:39 AM

6:06:24 AM – The absolute reality of this sequential left brain education is a child does not have a fully developed mind at the age when they start school and even before they reach the age of 12 they have had years of this sequential conditioning and so their mind never even matures because it is thrown into the left brain state, so a person never even gets a chance to achieve a mature balanced mind.

The mind is simply conditioned into this extreme left brain state before it even matures so a person never gets to feel what a balanced mind even feels like so they perceive their mind is normal simply because they never felt a normal mind because they were conditioned at such a young age. Do you understand why Abraham and Lot burned your dam cities to the ground? Do you understand why I do not find fault with what they did to the sane? Do you understand anything at all? I haven't slept for a while so I submit I am sloppy but I get this weird impression I can't reach you at all. I say tomato and you hear potato.- 6:14:09 AM

10:02:31 AM – Since I can't sleep and I am sloppy, so I will mumble to myself since the sane cannot understand anything I say ever. The darkness has a strong sense of time and that drives it mad. It is always impatient and always looking at the clock because time is real to it and that drives it mad. The darkness has to eat three times a day because it can never satisfy its hunger and so it eats itself to death and its hunger is never quenched. The darkness drinks itself to death because it gets drunk but cannot stay drunk so it has to keep getting high to make the sense of time less noticeable.

The darkness can never be satisfied with material things so it keeps taking more of them in a vain attempt to reach satisfaction and it never can reach satisfaction and it's sense of time is strong so that also drives it mad. The darkness tries many methods to escape its strong sense of time but it cannot escape itself. The darkness cannot escape its own fruits. The darkness see's all blessings as curses and all curses as blessings. The darkness is so dark it always sees the light as darkness and always sees itself as light. The darkness is a tormented beast that has no ability to escape itself. The sound of the clock ticking drives it mad.

The sound of its stomach growling drives it mad. The sound of the money clanging drives it mad. The sound of its heart beating makes it sad. - 10:14:03 AM

10:09:29 PM – I ate some pork chops in hopes it would make me forget what I understand and in hopes it would get me out of this infinite poorly disguised dairies fiasco, to no avail. Then it occurred to me the suggestion about do not eat unclean beasts or pigs. That is a nice way of saying do not associate with the ways of the sane because they are unclean beasts.

This is a good example of trying to communicate complexity to a being that has their right brain which deals with complexity veiled. They are simpleminded so they cannot grasp complexity so they take everything on face value because they have no choice.

So I will break it down.

A pig is a glutton.

Why is a glutton an unclean beast?

Because they got the education and thus are conditioned to extreme left brain and so they exhibit behavior relative to being physically focused as opposed to cerebrally focused because they never applied the fear not remedy or where simply never told it. They exhibit what are known as the seven deadly sins in their mindset or psychology.

So this is what an unclean beast is: [Genesis 3:14 ... cursed above all cattle, and above every beast of the field;...]

So what is an unclean beast?

A person who gets the education and is mentally unsound and that denotes they have a lot of fear because the Hypothalamus is not working properly in their unsound mental state among other things.

[2 Timothy 1:7 For God hath not given us the spirit of fear; but of power, and of love, and of a sound mind.]

This is all relative to fasting. A person of unsound mind will dread the prospect of fasting and one who has applied the fear not remedy will not even blink at that prospect because their minds do not even acknowledge hunger. To clarify that, a person who applies the remedy to the full measure does not even feel weak if they do not eat in 24 hours and their stomach does not growl and they do not have trouble thinking.

So fasting itself is a test to see who the unclean beast are and who are the ones who have applied fear not, submit to fear or , those who lose their life(mentally) preserve it. The reality is a glutton cannot go very long without food before they start showing symptoms and these symptoms are mental symptoms they are mentally unsound from the education.

So the comment about do not eat pigs they are unclean beasts has nothing to do with physical based ideals as the sane always assume everything is because that is their nature, but it is about a cerebral aspect. The ones who get the education are cursed above cattle mentally and that includes pigs also, so a pig is not an unclean beast in contrast to the ones who are cursed. They are cursed above all other creatures [Genesis 3:14 ... cursed above all cattle, and above every beast of the field;...] because their minds are so far in left brain from the education they are factually not really human beings mentally any longer , they are men.

[Genesis 11:5 And the LORD came down to see the city and the tower, which the children of men builded.]

206

The men are the unclean beasts and they educate their first born with the demotic and then make their own children build their vain towers to heaven called cities. In relation to the strong hunger, the mind itself is hindered from the education so the mind is at a disadvantage to begin with, in this extreme left brain state, one cannot think clearly even on a full stomach so it has this constant desire to eat so it can at least be at full capacity, so the body can operate in this unsound state of mind.

So the sane go a few hours without food and they cannot concentrate and they get physically weak because in reality their mind is so unbalance they are nearly brain dead. The complex powerhouse which is right brain is veiled to near silence and so they can only rely on the slothful simpleminded left brain to run the whole show and they cannot do it unless they have lots of food all the time. Three big meals a day are a symptom of gluttony and that is abnormal.

So this creates a big food shortage, and also they tend to get fat, and also they eat up everything and need large quantities of food, so after the written language was created they started growing crops because they could no longer live of the naturally growing food supply.

In relation to this [Genesis 3:14 … cursed… above every beast of the field;…] A wild pig can live easily in a natural surrounding and never need assistance. The sane have to actually go to survival classes to learn how live in a natural setting and they cannot live in that setting for long because their full mental capacity is long gone. They are only using the left hemisphere and that is the retarded hemisphere in contrast to the right hemisphere so the vanity is, the sane get the education and then have to get educated on how to live off the land when they should be able to live off the land unassisted to begin with, if they did not get the sequential education.

So the sane create all the problems and try to solve the problems but since they are mentally unsound they only create more problems. It is a self perpetuating downward spiral into extinction. Simply put: nature weeds out the unviable creatures one way or another. Once the mind of any creature is altered so far out of harmony they are running off the cliff of extinction and that is nature's solution to disharmony. The sane cannot figure out why everything is going south because they do not have the mental faculties to figure that obvious reality out. The sane veiled their mental complexity and continue to veil the next generations mental complexity so the whole boat is sinking and none of them will even think that until the boat goes under the waves. The fruits of the tree are all rotten because the tree /mind itself is conditioned to be rotten from about the age of seven by this invention, that is suppose to make one wise but in absolute reality is makes one retarded mentally unless the fear not remedy is applied, and that is nearly impossible because their hypothalamus is operating so poorly they are scared and nervous wrecks so they will not apply the fear not remedy. The tree of knowledge was fatal it's just a prolonged death rattle. - 11:36:25 AM

9/27/2009 4:59:26 PM – Pondering a judgment often is better than making one often.

Pondering a judgment, often is better than making one, often.
Pondering a judgment often, is better than making one often.
Pondering judgment often is better than making one, often.

6:17:30 PM - The one world order and one world currency concept is viable but the absolute freedom of speech and absolute right to bear arms must be maintained in order to achieve a checks and balance. This would mean any country that does not have absolute freedom of speech and absolute right to bear arms would have to adopt those principles to join this one world order and then there would be a universal consistency without the need to wage war to allow these basic human rights. Without absolute freedom of speech there is always going to be problems because once in a while someone comes along that has something worth listening to, and absolute freedom to bear arms ensures they are heard. There is always going to be a taskmaster that does not want his slaves to hear certain bits of information. Information like how the slaves can open their cages.- 6:26:09 PM

8:54:53 PM – Sacrifice a fatten calf.
[Sacrifice = Abraham and Isaac technique
Sacrifice = fear not
Sacrifice = [Luke 17:33 whosoever shall lose his life shall preserve it.]
Sacrifice = Submit
Sacrifice = No true philosopher fears death
Sacrifice = Sit in a cemetery alone at night and meditate.]

[Calf = Youth
Calf = [Genesis 3:14 … cursed above all cattle]]

[Fattened = Gluttony = seven deadly sins = mental symptoms of one in the left state of mind = physically focused instead of cerebrally focused.]

Fattened = [Genesis 3:14 … cursed… above every beast of the field;…]

Fattened calf = [1 Samuel 1:6 And her adversary also provoked her sore]

So sacrifice a fattened calf means one has to commit mental suicide. First thing is one has to understand the mind or the being.

X= the mind after it has been conditioned for many years into this left brain state by way or written language which is sequence based so one ends up mentally unsound and has lots of fear relative to [2 Timothy 1:7 For God hath not given us the spirit of fear; but of …. sound mind.]

[So, X = adversary and the adversary(alter ego) has to be sacrificed which is the fatten calf psychologically speaking.

Y = Sound mind where right and left hemisphere are working in harmony.]

So X + Sacrifice = Y

So one is conditioned as a child into the X state of mind and they have to sacrifice it or deny it to the extent the Y state of mind is restored. So Abraham took Isaac who represented a fattened calf or X and sacrificed him on the alter and then Isaac was mentally restored to Y state of mind.

So the X state of mind has to be ignored in a big way and the result will be the Y state of mind will be restored.

If one wants to look at it from a supernatural point of view. After one gets the education they exhibit symptoms of the devil and so they have to kill the devil or deny him and restore or unveil right brain/ the light.

If one wants to look at it from a psychological point of view one has to deny the Hypothalamus and that in turn shocks the mind back into mental harmony.

This requires self control from the being. So the being has two voices and they get to choose which one to listen to. In the X state of mind the fear voice is very loud and the no fear voice which is the

Y state of mind is very silent. So a person in the X state of mind is going to assume that fear voice is their conscience but it is not their true conscience is the Y no fear voice and it is very silent. This is why the center being or the core being has to understand that they have to go against the grain of the loud X voice and listen to the silenced voice of Y state of mind.

So in a scenario, an X person watches a scary movie and then goes in the bathroom and turns off the lights and looks into the mirror. Immediately that X state of mind is going to say "Turn on the lights or you will be harmed or killed." So the core being has to realize that is the X false voice and listen to the Y state of mind. There are many ways one can apply this method.

Saying the word perhaps often in fact is a form of sacrifice. If someone insults you and instead of attacking back you say Perhaps, you are sacrificing or submitting. This may actually be an effective method but perhaps it will not allow one to go the full measure in waking up.

Losing one's fear of death is the full measure. There cannot be any greater sacrifice than that. This is all in indication of how difficult it is to correct this left brain state the education puts one in. Simply put There is no substitute only varying degrees of correcting the left brain state to the [Luke 17:33 whosoever shall lose his life shall preserve it.] method.

So one has to literally love death when they are in the X brain state of mind. One has to find the most scary cemetery or crypt or mausoleum or abandoned house and make peace with their own sure death, and then go sit in that place alone with the understanding they are going to die.

This is what letting go means because it lets go of the X brain state and the Y brain state replaces it. One cannot go to a place they think they will live yet one does not want to jump into a frenzy of sharks either.

This is the sacrifice one has to make because they ate off the tree of knowledge. There is no substitute. Meditation and yoga and all the things may go part way but they will never take the place of the Abraham and Isaac method or the [Luke 17:33 whosoever shall lose his life shall preserve it.] or submit to death or , lose fear of death.

Everyone is going to wake up on their death bed anyway, but you can wake up and have a life and have many years of life before you die or you can wait until your death bed and have a few days of life. The reality is if you think you know what life is after you got all those years of left brain education and have not applied the fear not remedy you are infinitely mistaken. All one knows after they get all the left brain education is what mental death is like and what mental sorrow is like in contrast to how one feels after they apply the remedy. It is impossible one can know what mental life is because their mind never even developed before they were thrown into this sequential based education system, so they never even felt what normal mental function is ever like. They got robbed of mental function before mental function was even developed. The point being in order to jump from the physical based state of mind one is in after the education to the "cerebral" state of mind they have to use a cerebral method not a material method. -9:29:40 PM

It is done. Tis well.